Modern Marijuana Living

Modern Marijuana Living
Lighting the Way to a Healthy Lifestyle

Michael Green

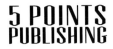
5 POINTS
PUBLISHING

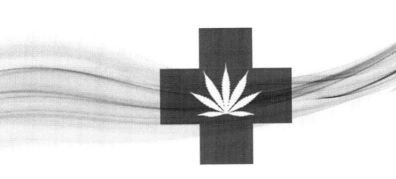

TABLE OF CONTENTS

Introduction 9

Chapter One: Getting Started. 13

Chapter Two: Every Day Is Judgment Day. 27

Chapter Three: Know Your Meds. 49

Chapter Four: Going Out into the World! 69

Chapter Five: Entertaining and the Marijuana Lifestyle 83

Chapter Six: Friends and Family and the Modern Toker 95

Chapter Seven: The Modern Marijuana User's Daily Guide . .103

Chapter Eight: Dating and Mary Jane .123

Chapter Nine: Travel and R&R. 131

Chapter Ten: Avoiding the Dark Side of the Smoke 141

Conclusion: Balancing the Mary Jane Life 159

Acknowledgments 165

About the Author 169

I dedicate this book to everyone who has ever
felt unfairly misrepresented by the ignorance,
the stigmas, or the negative stereotypes that have
been perpetuated since the days of
"Reefer Madness" and the "Slacker Stoner."
It is my sincere hope that these papers will help
us all find a cure.

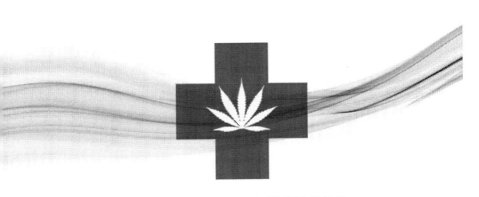

INTRODUCTION

U sing marijuana involves a lifestyle far more diverse than the negative picture commonly painted for the general public. Do you often wonder why using a medicinal herb with no known harmful side effects in place of pills pushed by giant pharmaceutical corporations, or "big pharma", (well-known for putting profit before patient health) is a *bad* thing? Why are we, who choose this herb, being stereotyped and stigmatized for making better and safer decisions for ourselves? Unfortunately, the "bad apples" have ruined responsible users' image far too long.

- *Are you tired of being referred to as the "Cheech" or "Chong" of your group of friends?*
- *Are you tired of not being taken seriously because you choose to use a plant for medicinal purposes?*
- *Are you tired of being stigmatized for choosing a safer*

*recreational alternative to any known drug, including
alcohol or tobacco?*

• *Are you tired of being constantly judged or criticized for
making an informed decision to choose marijuana to
treat a variety of ailments over pharmaceuticals?*

Well, it stops now! Many entertainers have sold out, exploiting the stigmatized aspects of marijuana, just to make a buck, ultimately feeding misinformation that discredits what is actually a much larger, more educated user base. Marijuana users are tired of being judged in such a negative light despite the fact that many are knowledgeable consumers and have been some of the greatest thinkers in our society, past and present, including Sir Richard Branson, Bill Gates, Steve Jobs, Stephen King, Queen Victoria, Carl Sagan, Ted Turner and George Washington, to name a few.

Early in my life, I majored in criminology at John Jay College of Criminal Justice with a plan on going into federal law enforcement. I've managed NYC bars and restaurants and have seen first-hand the significant differences between the marijuana and alcohol world. For many years, I established start-ups in non-marijuana related fields before realizing how much more passion and potential the marijuana industry held for me. I currently own and operate a successful medical marijuana dispensary in Los Angeles along with multiple marijuana news, media, and information web properties. I managed to accomplish all of this while maintaining a more than average daily marijuana use.

Modern Marijuana Living represents the *real marijuana user* of today, who is compassionate, intelligent, creative, stylish and when necessary—*very responsible and professional.* Throughout this book, I will offer a lot of valuable information, practical tips, and fresh concepts to help you avoid letting the plant you love get in the way of the other things you do in your life. I understand that trying to navigate the ever-changing and sometimes unfamiliar path to the American dream is growing more and more difficult. That's why it's important not to add to that struggle and put unnecessary obstacles in your way. Together, we can shed a clear light on nearly a century of misinformation, knock down the stigmas and stereotypes built up, and reinforced from the cynical exploitation, ignorant hysteria and selling out of the old cannabis era.

I contend that it's time for the new evolution of the modern day marijuana user's image from a "Cheech and Chong" couch potato slacker to a high-functioning, informed and sophisticated member of society. It's time to demand and uphold a new standard of excellence from today's marijuana culture and to establish a responsible code of behavior, knowledge and understanding for all.

—*Michael Green, Los Angeles, 2014*

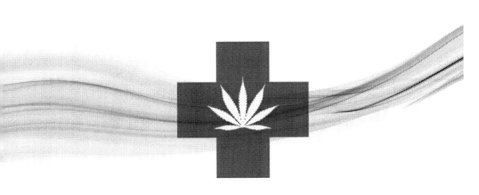

CHAPTER 1

GETTING STARTED

It's very important that the modern marijuana user should know the past history *and* current events of marijuana along with the social rules and personal habits necessary to responsibly "represent" today's marijuana culture. You should always be able to speak intelligently in defense of yourself and your fellow stoners against the continuous, unfair criticism and misrepresentation by conservative and ignorant factions in our society. We'll begin our journey along the path to a healthy marijuana lifestyle by discussing proper etiquette in three categories:

1. Smoking for the first time
2. The seasoned, but maybe poorly-mannered smoker
3. How to introduce someone to marijuana

Smoking for the First Time

Whether it's been a long road leading up to the moment or it happens in an instant of spontaneity, the first time you use marijuana can seem daunting for a variety of reasons. Of course, there are those of us who are natural explorers and are more likely to find that marijuana enters our lives sooner rather than later. But for others, from a very early age the plant may well have been systematically demonized through fear-mongering or powerful misinformation campaigns by their parents, teachers, or local law enforcement authorities. It's totally understandable that these tactics may have deterred them from even trying it.

In your parents' and fellow citizens' defense, there have been billions of taxpayer dollars spent on the war on drugs, creating fear, distrust and misinformation. We must start asking, "Why?" Why is marijuana (which in reality is a "miracle" plant) classified as a Schedule I drug and considered more dangerous than cocaine, which actually has less medicinal benefits? It's only when you begin to see who *really* benefits from all of this propaganda on a corporate and political level that it ever really begins to make sense. This categorization has effectively banned marijuana from being studied legally in order to prove its medicinal benefits. As legalization continues to be debated, reclassification on a federal level would not only recognize the medicinal benefits of marijuana, but it would also be much easier to implement lesser penalties. This move would bring about the de-criminalization of those seeking it out, possessing and/or distributing it and open it up for more scientific research to ensure we are able to maximize its potential and prove on the books marijuana's medicinal value. It's the next best thing to legalization, and is long overdue.

So you've done your research and are ready—or feel you, or someone you know may be ready—to jump into that sweet-smelling circle for the first go-round. Here are a few good things to know so you can keep your cool about you and not make a party foul.

It's good to know...
The most powerful tool that gets awakened
when you use marijuana is your mind.

Before even taking your first hit, take comfort in knowing that *no one has ever over-dosed and died from marijuana*. No matter how much you smoke or feel convinced at the time, you won't be poisoned from a marijuana edible (unless the other ingredients are bad) and you won't have an out-of-body experience or end up with permanent paralysis. However, sometimes a marijuana high can be a little difficult to control in the beginning. The sensation can run rampant on your senses and make you somewhat disoriented. You'll have a very low tolerance for the herb when beginning to use marijuana for the first time, and one hit could make you far higher than the effects of even a whole joint or multiple large bong hits for a seasoned marijuana user. While marijuana tolerance does work like alcohol in the sense that it does go up in time, even seasoned smokers can see a drastic reduction in their tolerance levels by switching strains regularly and or even taking short 1-3 day breaks.

Keep in mind that in today's world, depending on where you live, you may have other methods available to you for ingestion other than just smoking. Edibles, or vaporization, which is a smokeless and more potent form of using marijuana, can make you a more clean-smoking, healthier marijuana user. By choosing these methods, you eliminate the crude toxins of burnt plant material from entering your lungs, and on the most miniscule level, trace amounts of the butane from the lighter that you ingest every time you take a toke. It's also important to know that when you burn marijuana as opposed to vaporizing it, you can lose approximately 50% of its potency. That's reason enough to switch—if not for the long-term health benefits! If you've researched vaporizers, you know they can be expensive, but if you find the right one, it can save your life. Although we're finding out every day that the long and short term benefits of marijuana are mounting, you don't have to be a doctor or a heavy daily user to realize that something good is *not* happening to our lungs. The most you'll spend on a top of the line vaporizer now is $600. Would you rather spend dramatically more on medical bills later from smoke-related illness?

While this may seem like a lot of information to learn before you even take your first hit, it's best to form the healthiest habit possible from Day 1—or you should at least be given the opportunity to choose. If you're just beginning, knowing this information can save you from a potential lifetime of toxins. Take the time to educate yourself and experience healthier and more enjoyable for you and those around you.

Now that you've decided how you want to begin the exploration of marijuana, it's time to either go it alone, try it with a loved one, or delve in with a group of friends. A common side effect from first time use in groups or with others is paranoia, which generally feeds on pre-existing insecurities in the mind. One advantage of trying marijuana by yourself is that you can avoid the possibility of that kind of group experience, although smoking with *the right person in the right setting* can be the more enjoyable experience in many rewarding ways. Whichever way you decide to start, you should try to be in a very comfortable setting, if possible. Of course, sometimes social settings don't allow this and you'll have to compromise. This scenario is fine; but again, it's better for you to be cautious about trying it for the *first* time in a group situation.

If you follow the rules below, you're sure to begin your marijuana journey on a healthy and happy foot!

Ten Rules for the Beginner

1. ***Don't try and compete with seasoned smokers.*** It'll most likely be very entertaining and fun for them but it'll probably ruin the experience for you. Try one puff, inhale, and hold in as long as you can, then exhale and wait a good five minutes. *Only* if and when you feel like you're not feeling much of anything should you go for another hit. I know

it may be tempting when you see all the fun and exotic things your seasoned smoker pals are doing like bong hits, shotties, gravity bongs, "ghosting" hit after hit, etc., but don't worry, with your beginner's tolerance, you're getting the same effect from just one or two hits and, most likely your high will last much longer as well!

2. ***Don't try an edible as your first time.*** Depending on what products are available under current laws in your state, this tip cannot be stressed enough! Due to different body types, the effect and rate at which people metabolize marijuana can vary dramatically. It also can affect you in unpredictable waves and sometimes when people are unfamiliar with these psychoactive effects, they can become nauseous and/or be very anxious that the experience will never end. It's best to get an idea of how smoking or vaping marijuana affects you before trying an edible. When you're ready, edibles open up an amazing, healthier new world in marijuana use that is constantly evolving, thanks to science and the creativity of young entrepreneurs and businessmen entering the field.

3. ***When you're passed a joint or blunt, you must always be polite.*** First, thank the person handing it to you, then allow yourself a short time to take two inhales or "hits." Be sure to have time to hold the smoke in, but too much time may be deemed *"camping"* with the joint or blunt in hand. *"Camping" is considered very offensive or rude, especially if you aren't the one providing the marijuana.* "Bogart-ing" is another common

term used to describe "camping." This is in reference to the last name of famous actor Humphrey Bogart, who was commonly depicted with a cigarette always in the corner of his mouth, never seeming to actually draw or puff on it. *Note: If it's your first time, one inhale is recommended.* Kindly let the next person know you will only need one hit since it is your first time, so that they won't be confused as to whether or not proper smoking etiquette is still intact. Generally, stoner etiquette dictates passing to left, however the real importance is keeping the proper flow in whichever direction the grass is going.

4. *Be sure not to leave excess saliva on the end of the joint or blunt* so others may enjoy the same smoke without having to deal with the saliva of others. This rule *also* applies to lipstick and especially sticky lip-gloss!

5. *A properly rolled joint or blunt doesn't need to be pulled on extremely hard to get one large hit.* This ruins the joint or blunt by causing it to canoe. As a result, the other smokers can't get proper hits. It also dramatically shortens the lifespan of the joint. Needless to say, that can really mess up the evening of your fellow stoners, and we never want to do that!

6. *Don't allow the marijuana joint to go out while you are talking.* It's nice that you've finally gotten your chance, but there are others in the circle who may—believe it or not—be hanging more onto when you're going to pass that joint you're holding rather than onto your every word. Make

sure *everyone* is medicated in a timely manner so that more important things, such as stimulating conversation, can be enjoyed.

7. *When passed a bowl or large bong, be sure to only burn a partial section of fresh greens no matter how small, always leaving some green for the next person.* If this courtesy is impossible, be sure to give notice to the next person that it's likely that there's nothing left. (Knowing what we know now about smoking versus vaporization, it's considered very rude to give someone a burnt bowl to smoke).

8. *Avoid becoming a "Cookie Monster."* Resist the urge to let your uncontrollable munchies drive you to raid the food pantry, cupboards, or fridge of your host. Come prepared with your favorite drink and favorite snack. In fact—bring enough to share, and if possible, bring a small offering of your host's favorite snack.

9. *Always refrain from making a scene or drawing further attention to you or to the group.* If at any time you're feeling uncomfortable, just quietly excuse yourself to get some air.

10. *Don't put your friends in a difficult position when attempting to use marijuana for the first time.* It's common for many people to suffer a form of nausea or some increased unpleasant effects from marijuana if it's combined with light or heavy amounts of alcohol. Even longtime heavy users can still have that happen on occasion. You may or may not be one of these people, but it's recommended that for the first time *only try marijuana with no other drugs or*

alcohol in your system to truly see how it affects your body. Many people have had their first experience ruined due to the fact they experienced undesirable and unpleasant effects after mixing these two. As a result they were so put off, they never tried it again. Don't let this happen to you!

Here are some tips for the seasoned toker. Even if you've been at it for a while, you can add a little "class to your grass" etiquette, or at least check out this refresher list:

Ten Tips for the Seasoned Toker

1. *Always take only two hits, then pass.* Never try the "puff, puff, puff, puff, puff.... oh wait, that's only one hit technique."
2. *Always get the marijuana to other fellow smokers at their earliest convenience.*
3. *Never leave excess saliva on the end of joint blunt bowl or bong.*
4. *Patiently wait your turn.* But if it's necessary, kindly remind others of proper smoking etiquette.
5. *Never criticize the quality of marijuana provided if you didn't bring any yourself.*
6. *Never criticize the rolling or packing job of the blunt if you haven't rolled anything.*
7. *Always offer to help with the cost of the marijuana.* If that's just not possible, try and provide another item to make the smoking experience more enjoyable (for example, stimulating conversation and companionship, at the very least).
8. *Never canoe the joint.* An experienced toker understands they're responsible for stopping a "canoe in progress,"

usually by implementing the "lick finger to paper technique." Simply lick the tip of your finger and blot the part of the joint that is burning unevenly to allow the "cherry" to catch up and restore an even burn.

9. *Always leave some green for the next individual or alert them when the bowl or bong is empty.* When using edibles, make sure there's an even amount to go around according to tolerance levels.

10. *When lighting a blunt, be sure to take your time and pay attention to the task at hand.* The slightest mistake can ruin a perfectly rolled joint.

Introducing Marijuana to Others for the First Time

Now that you've found your love and enjoyment for marijuana, met someone in your life you want to share it with, or have a friend who's introduced you to "Mary Jane," it's very important that you make sure that you're a positive advocate and influence for marijuana. It begins with where we started. First and foremost, being educated on the subject should allow you to put anyone's mind at ease. *Marijuana is safer and effective in many medical and recreational ways.* We see what the mainstream media and certain religious and political forces want to do with marijuana, so it's up to us to usher in a new, more enlightened generation of responsible, educated marijuana users.

Many people say peer pressure is one of the leading causes of smoking marijuana for both teens and adults. I would like to introduce a new concept to those out there discussing marijuana with their friends or family: peer pressure may actually be *bad* for marijuana. As we discussed earlier, many people are deterred from marijuana use or even its basic acceptance largely due to the propaganda and misinformation generated not only from authorities, but also from common stigmas often perpetuated by the mainstream media. Through the years, stoner films depicted marijuana users as typically unmotivated slackers, munchies-consuming slobs, or simply dim-witted and unintelligent. There are overwhelming statistics supporting the contrary, and we all know these classic descriptions aren't true for the majority of users. However, when the herb is abused or mishandled, certain elements of those stigmas may *feel* true for some people when first trying marijuana—especially if they're not properly introduced to the marijuana culture.

Always focus on the enjoyment of the other people using the marijuana plant and with making sure they only have a positive experience. You should never put your fellow toker in an uncomfortable state where they can be ridiculed or be used for the amusement of others. It's understandable and quite common for someone to be so excited to share the plant with another, that certain things may be unintentionally forgotten. Unfortunately, that can be to the disadvantage of the person you want to introduce it to.

Here are a few tips to remember when introducing marijuana to a friend so that peer pressure doesn't ruin the experience:

1. *People's tolerance levels can be very different; therefore you must be respectful and knowledgeable of others and where they are on their marijuana journey.* Remember, it doesn't matter how that huge bong hit or that large volcano bag hit affects you, your newbie companion is just at the very beginning and will have a different reaction.

2. *Always patiently explain how to do even the simplest pot-related things, because common stoner terminology and techniques will be unfamiliar to the newbie.* First time usage can make someone feel nervous or anxious if they're unsure of how to properly act in the situation.

3. *Never ridicule or embarrass a newbie's first time unless it's in good fun and the person is in on the joke.* You never want to ruin someone's possible lifetime relationship with marijuana simply because it made you laugh in the moment.

4. *Make sure to keep your guest hydrated at the minimum and offer snacks and/or a place to rest after first time introduction.* It may not be completely necessary, but you should always be prepared.

5. *Always explain that there are many different types of marijuana.* If one strain doesn't work for them, they shouldn't give up; they should try other strains to be sure that marijuana is indeed not for them. There are many different strains and they all affect individuals differently; and while you can't provide all of these smoke options, at the minimum it's important to let them know there *are* other options.

6. *Always be respectful of those who do not enjoy marijuana as you do.* When someone says they've had enough or would like to pass, *never push.* Remain respectful of your guest's wishes.

As many of us marijuana users all over world have already discovered and continue to learn on a daily basis, the introduction of cannabis into someone's life can be life changing. It's a very real responsibility, but should also be a great joy to share with others. The information provided in these pages should help you to become a more informed marijuana user able to safely and comfortably bring this plant into the lives of others. At the very least, it'll make you a pleasure to share a bud with.

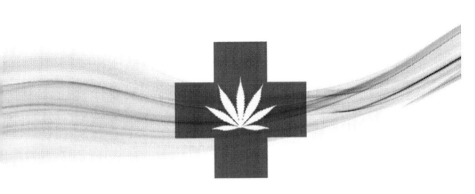

CHAPTER 2

EVERY DAY IS JUDGMENT DAY

*A modern marijuana consumer demands
to be taken seriously, and not be constantly
judged for the plant they use. You don't
buy into the BS, and do your best to lead
by example and read between the lines.*

Like it or not, marijuana has been attacked for nearly a century through propaganda, political lobbyists, and misguided activists or entertainers, with its users depicted as dirty, lazy, unintelligent, spaced out, and pretty much useless to society. Too often for a quick buck, marijuana has been trivialized and demeaned by the image of the classic stoner marijuana user. But, many other "greed over weed" variables have also contributed to the stigma of the "stoner" stereotypes that have thrived, in stark contrast to the responsible characteristics of the majority of its demographic. So what can we do? How can we avoid the very real concern and possibility that enjoying this wonderful plant could sabotage us in our personal, professional, and social lives?

We're committed to holding on tight to our marijuana culture, but others around us are simply not as informed as to all the benefits the plant truly has to offer. But this isn't about pleasing people. This is about how to avoid your bright potential from being blindly rejected and cast aside by the prejudgment of others simply because traces of your marijuana use can be detected. I'm not saying that this judgment is correct; I'm simply saying you need to understand the complex layers of the industry and realize that these negative images have been created and promoted by intelligent design. And above all, you must work harder not to give them more power by fueling them with your actions.

So what are your options? Well, you can say, "F- it, I'll wear what I want, talk how I want, do what I want…" and rebel your heart out to make your point. It's certainly been done over and over throughout time. And look, you're not wrong—you *can* and *should* be able to wear whatever you want, but in all reality in today's world, if you act and dress certain ways—like it or not, it can really set you back. *There's a time and a place for everything.* This chapter is meant to help you avoid being typecast before you ever even open your mouth, and when you do communicate, how to be taken seriously.

Part 1

A Dose of Prevention Can Prevent
a Lifetime of Negativity

I'm not trying to change who you are or how you dress, but it's
vital to understand the true nature and history of marijuana
and how important the role is today in changing the way marijuana users are viewed at large. He/she understands that regardless of how perfectly logical the argument is for legalizing
marijuana on a medicinal and economic level, there are other,
more selfish and cynical motives being served. *Who is profiting
by keeping marijuana illegal?* Ultimately, you must understand
that many people will do everything they can, for as long as
they can, to discredit marijuana users because it benefits them.
These powerful and influential detractors have set clever traps
to further their cause such as taking the distinctive clothing
styles and colorful gear marijuana users favor and encouraging
mainstream America to associate those items with an unclean,
unmotivated individual. Yes, these traps can be unfair because
hoodies, flip-flops, and sweatpants are *really* comfortable *all* the
time, but if you ever want to move forward in the real world
we live in today—if only to empower yourself to make a bigger difference later (and that goes for the marijuana industry
also!)—you have to "play the game" to avoid these traps starting right now. A *major part of the game is to avoid putting unnecessary obstacles in your way.*

Sometimes, marijuana can influence the way you look, act,

and talk without you realizing it. While usually pot is used to help inspire creativity and identify your own style, it can also lead to some undesirable characteristics popping up in your everyday appearance, behavior, and speech. In the second part of this chapter we're gong to address these issues in more detail, focusing on how to win the respect of your peers and colleagues, all while maintaining your mild-to-heavy daily marijuana intake.

Part 2
You Can't Win the War without First Winning Many Battles

General Appearance

Don't let "expressing yourself" mean "letting yourself go." Even the "messy look" needs proper maintenance. Consistent showering and even light grooming can be the fine line between the "longhaired, bearded, dirty, smelly, homeless hippy" and the "suave, sophisticated, free-spirited genius-philosopher, but just misunderstood" look. Seriously, a little goes a long way here, and for men, basic upkeep comes from investing in an electric razor or even some cheap disposables if necessary. You need to always understand the value of being well groomed—or at least stylishly unkempt.

Women who apply makeup on a regular basis should consider applying makeup *before* "toking" to prevent over-obsessing in the mirror (this applies to hairstyling as well). It's usually best to add eye-drops *before* applying mascara if you plan on toking *after* and want to hide the redness.

Dreadlocks Are Cool

Just be prepared: You won't be taken seriously and you'll always be associated with smoking and da-Ganja regardless of your many other great qualities. It's not the fault of the public for making these judgments, but you owe it to yourself not to be negatively branded in such a manner as not to overshadow your other great qualities—unless you believe that dreadlocks benefit you or you have them for religious reasons. *You* may think your "Ganja" style is simply a fashion statement, but to *everyone* else it screams pothead, and, of course, you never want to be referred to in a negative light.

Posture

It's very good to be aware of your posture for its variety of benefits. Many people use marijuana to treat chronic pain, which is generally brought on by bad posture. One preventive measure in pain management could just be correcting your posture. "Sit up straight!" That common reminder can be so annoying! Our parents always correct us, our partners constantly urge us, and old-timers randomly warn us that we'll "regret it later in life…" Well, have you ever looked at yourself in a video and noticed how your posture can set you apart, even in a crowd? Slouching and bad posture are usually associated with bad manners or a "less together" individual. It's a constant battle for me as well, but by working on your posture you can really save your body a lot of stress and make yourself look as natural as possible while projecting a stronger presence that exudes confidence. Confidence can unlock any avenue for success. So, *sit up straight for* a start—or you can just stay annoyed, form painful, life-long spine and neck problems, and look like "Quasimodo" or "Lurch" from *The Addams Family.* It seems like self-sabotage to literally diminish your image because these words of wisdom are "annoying" to you.

Yoga can go a long way in correcting bad posture and restoring core strength. The fairer sex seems to already be aware of this phenomenon. But for some reason, yoga typically has a negative image for many straight men. Right? Well, if being around the ladies stretching in yoga pants while making myself healthier, in good shape, and thus better equipped to please them is *lame,* then maybe we men should ask ourselves, who decides what is taboo or not? A real man should be prepared to risk a little razzing by some buddies at the expense of being more enlightened and leading by example. At the end of the day, would you rather be the uneducated, stiff old man dying slowly in agony like many of our ancestors did, or the man who takes advantage of a free, widely used exercise form that's known to increase longevity and provide a much higher quality of life in your twilight years? Who you will be in the future is defined by the decisions you make today. Sometimes, just because an idea is popular, it is planted to the disadvantage of the common man, so you must always look at certain taboos in society and other subjects with an open mind and attempt to make your own *informed* decisions.

Choosing What to Wear

There's a right time and place for everything. We all love our favorite everyday jeans for casual wear, but when we have to dress up, whether for a family function or a job interview, clean clothes that are fresh smelling and wrinkle-free go a long way. For starters, do regular laundry and keep your clothes relatively clean. You're already at an unfair disadvantage due to the continual misrepresentation of marijuana smokers for generations through exaggerated, almost cartoonish images and characterizations in books, TV, and film, coupled with some highly publicized "bad stoner apples" in real life. Remember: others are judging your appearance and you must try harder to make others around you more comfortable—not only for them, but ultimately, for yourself. Pick and choose your battles in this area and consider this: when you've been battling your parents/roommates/partner on and off about your marijuana use and all the styles they don't approve of or understand to the point that they just don't know what do to anymore, the reality is, more than half the time *they* just don't want be embarrassed and/or look bad in front of their friends and colleagues. On the flip side, *you* really just want them to get off your back, so maybe if you just played the game—even a little compromise with them—they'll give you a break, too. Just make them look like the parent they want to be in front of their friends and they'll probably leave you alone the rest of the time. It's worth trying no matter how stubborn you are, how petty and ridiculous you think it all is or how determined you are to make a sartorial stand. In this situation, you're not really giving in; you're just graduating from the game of checkers to chess.

What you choose to wear day-to-day and the little things you choose to highlight in your appearance is your decision. But if you want to avoid being negatively judged as an old-time, cannabis era stoner, there are some types of clothing gear and accessories you can avoid or at least know the right time and place for them.

Clothing not to Wear to Avoid Marijuana Stereotypes: Tie-dye T-shirts

These iconic colorful T-shirts are fine to wear for a day of Frisbee on the beach, at a fresh meadow park, or a Coachella concert. Even a hippy-themed party would be a great place to wear it! Now, the tie-dye T-shirt is really just classic cool in general, but make no mistake, wearing one is like painting a giant marijuana/recreational psychedelic drug user bulls-eye on your back! Nothing wrong with it, but if you want to avoid being labeled with some stereotypes and wrong assumptions, maybe save the T for a suitable occasion like when you paint your house, watch a game or mow your lawn.

Everything Hemp / Hippy Style

The occasional hemp bracelet or necklace trinket can be cool and stylish. Even making clothes out of hemp can be a huge economical boost in a legalized world, but right now, you just look like a space cadet or an old-school unemployed hippy back from the commune. There's a right place and time for marijuana-related clothing and just because you believe in something, it doesn't mean you must become a human label for it at the expense of possibly not being taken seriously by people who can really help your cause to make a larger difference. Sometimes small sacrifices in personal preference must be made to lift the negative images associated with "the slacker" or "dirty" marijuana user.

Ladies, while letting your body hair grow wild may really make a "statement" and show your dedication to all things natural and organic, it's also a potential fast track straight to the "friend zone".

Hoodies All Day, Everyday

I love a hoodie as much as the next guy and it's a constant battle for me to leave it home, but when you have to get a job and make money, or try to raise money for an idea, a hoodie just doesn't get you there no matter how hip and cool you look. Why lower your odds of success so dramatically? Just put your hoodie on later when the business is done and you're celebrating your new job or investment in your own environment. Trust me, your comfy hoodie will still be waiting for you.

Pajama Clothes

I get it. You're so laid back and chill, you don't even need to get dressed in street clothes. Really? Well, to everyone else, since you're not Hugh Hefner, you probably don't look very reliable and most likely not the guy your friends will think to call in the future to start up a business or even brainstorm ideas with. But hey! You're expressing yourself! I can understand that, but life is one long journey and the choices we make now can and will have long-term effects on how we are perceived by others in the outside world.

Marijuana Gear/Stoner Memorabilia

We all like T-shirts with cool logos, and are always finding ways to express that we are 420 friendly in hopes of connecting with others. This gear may be fun for collecting or for sporting at marijuana related events, but in situations where you want or need to be taken more seriously in a professional setting or just to make a good impression with a friends or parents, these items should be the last things you choose as fashion or decorating options.

Things to Try and Prevent or Avoid from being Visible That Result from Heavy Marijuana Smoking

It's important to know that many of the following conditions or issues can completely be avoided by choosing edibles or vaporization as an alternative to smoking. While you should always try to "vape" while educating and informing others as to benefits of this, time and finances currently make household vaporizing largely unavailable to many of the marijuana users out there. For the majority of tokers out there still using more traditional methods of ingesting marijuana, here are a few tips to help keep whoever needs to be, kept off of your tracks:

- **Red Eyes:** While vaporization won't save you from this side effect and may increase it, carrying a form of red eye relief is imperative to maintain the appearance of clarity to people around you. This is essential to satisfy those who may otherwise unfairly judge you, your actions or expressions simply due to the fact that you show signs of marijuana use. Applying eye drops just prior to marijuana use and then again after—*if necessary*—is more effective at keeping the red out and helps prevent having to wait longer for the redness to go away naturally.

• **Resin stained lips and/or fingertips:** Believe it or not, that dark blemish on your lip that won't go away didn't just come out of nowhere. Newsflash: other people notice it too. We all love our own various ways of using marijuana, but some of the most common and more popular ways to use marijuana can unfortunately leave some undesirable side effects behind. Smoking lots of joints, blunts, and spliffs, typically leads to this particular problem. Either avoid these methods altogether or take small steps to prevent yourself from getting these undesirable stains on your lips and fingertips. For starters, simply try alternating sides of the lips between inhales and/or whole joints or blunts. Also, for health reasons, don't "pull" on the "roach" extremely hard, if at all. Most of the resin build-up is at the end of the joint or blunt and just gunks up the roach, so if you are always roasting the roach, you're more susceptible to these types of stains and/or heat damage on the throat. It's far healthier to save roaches and reroll them altogether. Not only that, but the next combination joint will be *extra* strong from all the resin build-up saved from previous smokes. *It's the heat from the joint that is truly the most harmful part for you.* By avoiding harsh heat on your throat, you're avoiding one of the negative side effects generally found from smoking. Washing your hands after smoking and a simple mirror smile check can avoid giving you away with your first smile or handshake. You can also avoid leaving trace elements of the strong aroma that resin can have in smaller amounts if stains are left unseen on your body or cloths, even stuck to your shoe.

- **Dark circles under the eyes:** Some people are born with these, but some people definitely get them *more* when they use marijuana. This is another plus for vaporization. Many kinds of smoke have toxins that can cause these shadowy rings. If you're someone who definitely notices an increase in dark circles/ pale skin/ poor circulation, many of these symptoms can be alleviated or avoided altogether by switching to safer forms of marijuana use such as vaporization for daily use, or edibles that are dosed to the necessary strength for the individual. You may spend an unquantifiable amount of your money on marijuana in a lifetime. How much would you spend on a device that could save your life, or at least, keep you healthier while at the same time delivering more potency and flavor out of the marijuana you have been smoking and all the bud you will smoke from this day forward. You're worth it! Believe me, it will only make you healthier and your marijuana experience more rewarding on multiple levels.

- **Oooohhh... That Smell:** Marijuana. This has been an ongoing task for marijuana smokers and closet cigarette smokers alike for years. While there are many methods for trying to mask the smell of the plant while you are smoking it and there are odorless edible marijuana products available, I'm going to discuss how to mask this telltale smell after use and how before going into public, you can keep your marijuana use under the radar.

Quick Tips to Masking the Smell

- **Brush your teeth:** Ideally you would brush your teeth and wash around your mouth (a lot of smell stays there, especially with that cool facial hair). After flossing, follow with a mint and or gum. Next, take some deep breaths to coat the throat and the airways from the lungs to the mouth with something nice. An unexpected cough while you're standing in a group will undoubtedly "freshen the air" with a strong whiff of your last toke and instantly give you up if you're not prepared. For ladies, a quick swipe of flavored lip balm will also help.

- **Wash your hands:** Most of the smell from smoking a joint can really stick to your fingers; I mean *really*. If you can't get access to a sink right away, as silly as it may seem, you may want to invest in a smoking glove. Even an old batting or golf glove would do the trick and enable ease of use while acting as a shield for your hand. Ideally, you could use a glove and wash afterwards.

- **Avoid taking the smell with you:** Marijuana smoke can get in your clothes and your hair. Men usually have shorter hair and often wear sports hats, so it's not as common a problem as it is for women. Clothing can be a vessel for that sweet smell to follow you everywhere your wardrobe does, so keep in mind to choose *fabric* fresheners over *air* fresheners. Let's start with the immediate smoking cover-up solution: It's good to try and smoke in ventilated areas if at all possible. "Hot boxing" (toking in an area that is sealed from ventilation, usually creating a thick smoky atmosphere) is the worst-case scenario, because by limiting the amount you smell in the beginning, you make the cover-up that much easier. If possible, wear a jacket or a wrap that you aren't going to wear out to act as shield for your "work" or "going out" clothes. If you can't take a smoking jacket with you (understandable), you may be wise to let yourself air out a little before heading indoors right away. At the least, you should have some kind of perfume or cologne, but don't go too crazy with atomizer because that can also be taken as a sign that you're trying to hide something and it will give you away. Using a satin hair cap will also protect your hair from becoming smelly before you go out. A small bottle of hand sanitizer can help a lot too, if you can't take steps to wash your hands as mentioned above.

The second problem you want to avoid can happen when you haven't even had anything to smoke that day or possibly for days! People often slowly introduce marijuana into their daily life without taking into consideration some of the little things they're bringing in as well. When it comes to household marijuana smoking, if you're doing it in your home (especially if not "vaping" or using edibles), your clothes are absorbing all of that smoke that dissipates every time you exhale, *if* your closet or storage area where you store jackets is in proximity to where you generally use marijuana. This occurs even if it's only connected by a hallway and open door. In these scenarios, door drafts are great to prevent smoke from entering into undesirable rooms, or worse, into the hallways in your apartment building. In other words, that perfect suit that you keep nice and crisp for that next big meeting is also getting nice and dank—ready to sabotage your deal before you even walk into the meeting. Or worse, it makes the wrong lasting impression as you give your girlfriend or boyfriend's mom a "sweet smelling" hug for the first time. Swearing that you didn't smoke before you came won't change anything. *The best weapon is always prevention.*

I have outlined the many ways to avoid sabotaging yourself with bad habits in this chapter. Armed with this valuable information, it's your duty to alert any other fellow marijuana users if you notice them faltering. You should always be trying to help create and maintain a positive image for marijuana users everywhere without negatively infringing on their rights to the freedom of expression.

Now that you've made all the necessary adjustments to your general appearance and are always aware of the right time and place for letting your "inner marijuana culture" shine through, remember: you'll be offered opportunities to contribute to society in powerful ways, not because you are *changing for them,* but because you are *empowering yourself!* So armed with your modern *anti-*stoner makeover, be sure not to backslide and let those common stoner language habits get in your way and ruin all the hard work you've done!

Part 3
Polishing Your Verbal Skills

The value in being able to communicate clearly and eloquently, and to draw on a good vocabulary that makes it possible to express your feelings intelligently in any situation, with any audience, is incalculable. You must master your expression if you want to gain the respect of others and speak intelligently on any subject—especially the subject of marijuana. Now, it's true that some people are more naturally gifted at articulation, but you don't have to be a great public speaker to command respect when you do speak. There are ways to strengthen these abilities by looking up words you don't know.

The Internet is an amazing tool that's virtually available everywhere. If it's too late for traditional school, just smoke a little and go online to look up some synonyms for some of the words you use in everyday conversation just to change it up a little. Being unable to express yourself clearly can be a major liability, considering that is the only way to convey your insights to others around you. Exercising these particular muscles and utilizing language-building skills will only empower you in anything you do.

Maybe get crazy and learn another language and just blow your friends', co-workers', and relatives' minds.

- **Articulation**: A dose of prevention can go a long way when it comes to avoiding cliché stoner terminology that was first made famous by old stoner comedies which have only fuelled the negative image of the messed up, irresponsible stoner for decades. Sure, some of them are funny, but they've given modern day marijuana users a bad name, and have created further barriers in the march towards legalization. By becoming more articulate, you'll keep the respect and interest of others while clearly and effectively expressing your own viewpoint in return. If you focus on speaking intelligently without peppering your speech with slang, bad grammar, and out-right swearing, all while maintaining eye contact (with the added confidence gotten from your red eye relief), you'll be sure to start commanding and charming all the members of your professional and/or philosophical smoking circles.

- **Stoner Lingo to Avoid:**
  You: "Hey Maaan, that's just way I talk... come on brah, you can't be serious!"
  Potential Employer: "Yeah sorry Brah, we just don't hire that way, but hey Maaaan, good luck with that."
  If you begin or end your sentence with any of these types of words: *dude/duuuude, man/maaaan, bro/brah, ummm/uuuhhh, like or "text speak" (omg/ lol) etc.,* you're basically implying that no one should take anything you say seriously—that you're talking like an classic uncouth, unprofessional stoner. In other words, you'd be pegged

as an unintelligent and unmotivated individual. It doesn't matter if it's generally not true, so stop giving them ammo and undermining yourself by falling into the bad habits of stoner lingo.

• **Tone:** Tone can be the simplest or most difficult thing to master, depending on the environment and/or strains smoked. Add emails and text messages to the mix and deciphering your genius wit from unintended cruel insults or rude, offensive remarks can get tricky. Not everyone can be in your head and know exactly how you mean things all the time. Tone can go far, not only to help others identify your mood, but to help you to command the conversation and relay your sincerity—or lack thereof—on the subject. There's a proper tone of voice for every situation, like knowing when to use your indoor and outdoor voices. You must always be very aware and diligent to use the proper tone in the right environment to achieve the maximum results. Look for the concept in everything as to gain deeper understanding, so that you can teach to others what you know if necessary. Here are a few ideas to conceptualize in order to fine-tune your articulation and tone:

• **Please and Thank You:** It would seem that these words have been lost on everyone—stoners and non-stoners alike. Believe me, these simple words can go a long way!

• **Less is More**: Sometimes, quietly observing and taking in your surroundings and other people's perspectives can offer you special insights that you may not have been able to make if you are too busy trying to be at the center of attention. Wait to say something insightful, think it out, and then articulate it clearly. *Always listen to others* if you expect the same in return. *Less is more!*

• **Take Notes:** We can all lose our train of thought once in awhile in this crazy world we live in, but obviously this can happen more when using marijuana, so it helps to take notes to organize your thoughts. This way, you can bail yourself out if you find yourself a little "spaced-out" in the middle of something important, like a speech or business meeting. If you're going to function as a high-level marijuana user, you need to always come prepared. You must take extra steps to not let marijuana become a negative force in the work environment, and at the very least, not give peers any reason to feel negative about your marijuana use. Try hard not to give marijuana users a bad name through poor representation.

In a perfect world, if you use slang or dirty language, you shouldn't have to change it for anyone.

But, the reality is, that if you want to get what you want and then keep it, you have to know when to turn it on and off. By limiting yourself to sloppy language only in your *off time*, you won't have to worry about being poor and unemployed *full time*. It's already tough enough to avoid unemployment in today's economy, even if you've got a college degree. Certainly the last thing you want to do is provide a reason to be "weeded" out from any type of selection process!

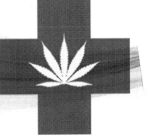

CHAPTER 3

KNOW YOUR MEDS

"The times, they are a' changing'"—Bob Dylan

The world of marijuana strains is evolving at an unprecedented rate in human history. Science has finally gotten more involved, not only domestically but internationally as well. What they are finding is constantly blowing the lids off of older myths and misinformation about marijuana strains that have been previously perpetuated through false studies and poor representations of marijuana from the "old cannabis era". Thankfully, we are able to correct many of the mistakes of the times through a little more thorough research and a better general outlook on the well being of fellow tokers.

To be an educated, health-conscious and responsible

rijuana user, you must at the very least be familiar with the different types of strains and their effects. The purpose of this chapter will be to focus on the different types of marijuana strains; however, it is important to understand that these are general guidelines and do not represent all the strains of the particular category. The most common types of marijuana strains are typically Sativa, Indica, or a Hybrid. CBD and the need for CBD strains (Cannibidiol: a non-psychoactive component of *marijuana* that possesses a wide range of therapeutic benefits) are important concepts for every serious stoner to understand.

The following is a short basic guide on each strain:

- **Sativa:** These are generally known as daytime use strains. The reason for this is that they typically provide a more *psychoactive* effect on the user rather than having a *heavy body effect* for the user, leaving their minds stimulated without the drag on the body. These are great for people with mood disorders, stress and anxiety. They typically help relieve these symptoms without leaving the user feeling tired or sluggish. Unfortunately, these strains usually don't help to alleviate physical pain and often, because of the increased psychoactive effects on the user, the sativa strains may exacerbate them, which may lead to increased agitation with the painful symptom.

- **Indica:** These strains are generally known for

providing a heavier effect on the body. The effects may range from minor pain relief, to the feeling of total paralysis (which, of course, has never physically happened, outside of the mind) and a wide spectrum in between. Appetite stimulation, nausea reduction, and sleep aid are just a few other things marijuana users get from these strains.

- **Hybrids:** Think of a mad scientist trying to create "custom strains": basically knowing what we know now about the main types of strains and their general effects on users, you can begin to understand where hybrids come from. When creating a hybrid, the scientist or grower must first identify the types of effects he would ideally want to produce with the strain. Once he has identified these traits, he can seek out strains that have them. When he's found a combination of the right types of strains, the scientist or grower can cross the genetics to try and take the ideal effects they find in the different types of strains and roll it all into one for you. Many times this can create much confusion for the buyer, simply due to the addition of so many new names to the market. It's impossible to keep up with all of the "Frankenstein" type creations of growers all over the country, all contributing to the confusion of the marijuana name game. Besides being a problem in itself, this leaves the consumer susceptible to certain exploitations that you should be sure to keep an eye out for.

• **CBD Heavy Strains:** One of the largest discoveries in the marijuana field has been in the effects of CBD. Basically, CBD helps with pain, inflammation, and often forms of anxiety. It's an anti-convulsant, anti-arthritic, and neuro-protective agent that doesn't induce psycho activity. Translation: this is the property found in marijuana responsible for your pain relief. When growers locked on the idea that it was only the THC that got you high, they tried to just breed more potent THC strains and slowly bred out much of the CBD. As we have learned more in recent years, growers have found that by doing the reverse and breeding high CBD/ low THC strains, they can effectively treat pain with little of the psychoactive or "getting high" effects. Many people prefer this if the psychoactive effects are generally too strong for them, but they still want the pain relief they find from that particular strain. On the contrary, if you find strains with high levels of THC *and* CBD, you will be in for one very strong experience.

This new modern research is yet another testament to the incompetence that defined the old stoner era. Back in the 60's and 70's, they believed that THC/TRICHOMES/ or the "pretty crystals" were the only things responsible for all the effects the user got from marijuana. In more recent years, now that science has been able to have a hand in culturing marijuana and people are questioning what has been relentlessly fed to them for decades, finally real light is beginning to be shed on the other components found throughout the marijuana plant and the effects. As I write this book, they number over 420!

• **The "Marijuana Name Game":** This has become one of the biggest and most confusing problems for the emerging marijuana industry. The core of the problem stems from poor documentation by growers, an inconsistent naming system and the abuse of marijuana sellers taking advantage of patients to move poor or recycled product under a new "cooler" name. Sometimes this week's new "Moonwalker" was last week's "Bubba Skywalker". To go even further, some growers will actually name different parts of the same plant to create the illusion to consumers that these are different strains. The reality is that it is the *same* strain but can look slightly different on different parts of the plant, and with excess product, there's a real temptation by the seller to change names. *Don't be a victim; inspect closely.* Understanding what we now know about hybrids, the crazy names of these strains today are largely based on the original *Indica* and *Sativa* strains that have very interesting names themselves. The result is a continual spawning of endless combinations of especially unique names.

- **Endless Strains for Endless Profit:** When you're standing in a collective gazing at a seemingly endless number of strains on display, always beware—there are still those who will aim to confuse the consumer to make a profit. Always beware of "special deals" and remember the old adage: If it seems too good to be true, usually it is. Many times in the medical and recreational marijuana market, we find ourselves faced with deals that are too good to be true. Keep in mind that there's usually a catch. When finding incredible marijuana deals, it's important to understand how marijuana makes its way into shops (if it's not grown by growers at the actual location you buy it). Some people take their marijuana business and growing operations very seriously, providing top-of-the-line marijuana. They're well funded and able to keep the quality control demanded by the current marijuana user base.

However, not everyone who enters the market is so inclined or willing to pay top dollar for their patient's strains. Many people can't afford the kinds of expensive and sophisticated setups necessary to enter the market at that level. Instead, they generally turn to what's called "gorilla growing", or "backpacking" on a farm or public land. The grower will throw down seeds illegally and come back at a later date to pick the plant when it's ready for harvest. Minimal investment is needed so that this type of marijuana crop can be sold back to the market for outrageously lower prices and still generate a profit for the grower. Of course, the quality of the product usually suffers dramatically. What most people don't think about is all of the chemicals and pesticides used by the farm that are also being sprayed on the marijuana plants. In most cases, information about all the toxins that have been added to the plants is never disclosed or is possibly not even known in depth by the grower. It's important to find a co-operative that's looking out for you and will make the effort to avoid these "special deals" and demand tested products for their user base. However, many of the fly-by night operations that are mostly responsible for a large amount of the marijuana distribution in medical marijuana states have this problem. These very shady places price-slash tainted goods to sell those "special deals" for the quick "turn-and-burn" because they know if you get sick or have a problem, there's no accountability. More than likely they'll be moving locations or disappearing with no paper trail in the very near future—just like the "broker" they most likely got it from. You must always be skeptical of seemingly amazing marijuana deals and remember: usually you get what you pay for. The real shame is that without proper and responsible oversight, many people who are now seeking out marijuana for medicinal use and being shamelessly ripped off are the ones who would be more susceptible to illness from these cheap tactics. Luckily, in a world of communication overload, we can try avoiding these kinds of places by word of mouth and utilizing some of the sites that review marijuana dispensaries. For now, you are your best protector!

• **Mind Over Strain:** The mind is the most incredible machine known to man in the universe. We're still only scratching the surface to understand the human brain's true potential and its ability to not only master and control your senses, but possibly its part in healing yourself in many ways as well. Sometimes getting too high allows our minds to play tricks on us. This often leads to paranoia and/or confusion. Maybe a little less THC is what you really need. Understanding the different combinations of THC and CBD available and the effects that those combinations have, can help you hone in on your ideal strains. This can make you a more effective host as well as give you your perfect effect for the right time of day.

"You can't always get what you *want*, but sometimes you get what you *need.*" Sometimes a strain just gives you exactly what you need. Some strains designed for sleep aid are effective day or night. *Not all strains affect everyone the same way, at the same time.* In fact, sometimes *the same strain can affect the same user different ways at different times.* For example: you decide to use a strong OG type of Indica strain for the first time. Maybe that time you have it and it's exactly what the doctor ordered— medicated pain relief, but not incapacitation etc., but the next time you use that same strain, it knocks you right out. Next thing you know, you're waking up at 3am on the couch with all the lights on, and something burning in the oven. WTF? Well generally, the simplest explanation is that *the plant usually gives us what we need.*

Consider this: in the first scenario, the individual may be well-rested and be in a recreational state of mind; therefore, what the body is needing is more *stress relief* as opposed to *rehabilitation*. In the second scenario, the individual may use this same strain when he's finally had a chance to get off his feet after a long hard day of work. He smokes a little bowl and is knocked right out. This may really not have anything to do with the strain; sometimes the body needs what it needs, whether it be nourishment (munchies), sleep, or pain relief. These effects generally manifest based on what the body needs. As I stated earlier, your mind can play tricks on itself, so it's important to get that under control so you can really begin to sort out what necessary effects you get from individual strains. This knowledge and understanding will ultimately make you an informed and educated consumer.

- **Being an Educated Consumer Can Make All the Difference:** The easy accessibility to a multitude of strains in legalized states makes marijuana selection like being a kid in a candy store, and while this probably sounds great to any stoner, remember, candy is a hell of a lot cheaper! Sorting through all the types of strains without really knowing the different effects can leave you not only spending an obscenely large amount of money, but also most likely being very frustrated at many of the strains' effects. There are different reasons why people like certain strains of marijuana, and they usually end up falling somewhere on the strain spectrum they can identify, whether it be with *Sativas, Indicas, or Hybrids.* You can dramatically narrow your options and at least begin to navigate your own strain preferences. Some people like marijuana to give them a creative feeling and some like it more to take them down a notch. There are all kinds of strains that can deliver both types of effects. The problem is, that if you are looking for one and get the other that leaves you unhappy and out-of-pocket a pretty penny.

Tolerance can be another factor here: No matter how great your favorite strain is, buying too much in bulk and only smoking it exclusively will build up your tolerance and dampen the effects over time. It's much better to split up that ounce that you're about to purchase. Get half of your favorite and maybe split the rest between a few new products similar to your favorite to help expand your horizon. This way you won't ruin your favorite strain by literally getting "burned out" on it.

Remember to always beware of incredible deals! You never want to be the recipient of "gorilla grown" marijuana. Typically in life, you get what you pay for, and it's no surprise to anyone that advice also applies to marijuana—shocker!

- **Variety Is the Spice of Life:** As you become more of a connoisseur about your strain use, you can begin to expand your daily arsenal of strains. There really is a right time and place for every strain, even if one strain has multiple times and places for it alone! There are tremendous advantages to knowing what strain is good for getting your day started and which one is a good night cap. Such knowledge ensures that you won't mix them up. Many new marijuana users fall into the trap of "strain ignorance." They want to smoke during the day, but either they only have certain types of heavier strains available to them or don't understand that not all weeds are the same and can have dramatically different effects on the user. It can mean all the difference between "waking and baking" while continuing on to tackle all of your day's projects enthusiastically, or wanting to just crawl back into bed, feeling unmotivated and unproductive (which can often carry over into the next day). You wouldn't take a sleeping pill before your big day would you? It's the same concept here. *Know the effects you're going to get beforehand to avoid ruining your day or even worse slipping into bad long-term habits of* *unproductivity.* Switching strains may just be the answer for those who find themselves with this problem.

- **To Grind or not to Grind?** This is a commonly debated question. Answer: Definitely Grind! But don't grind all of your marijuana right when you get it. Have you ever packed a bowl nice and fat with solid nugs only to wonder why it's so hard to hit and seems cashed right away? For years this has been the best way to waste marijuana and undermine the actual marijuana being smoked. By not grinding your weed, you are minimizing the surface area of the bud there is to burn and this doesn't allow you to get a very "milky" hit at all. Also, poor packing often leads to the clogging of the bowl. Depending on the different densities of the buds, you can go through a half gram at a time and hardly get the desired effects for one person let alone for a few people trying to share. By taking a few small steps, you can really unlock the ultimate potential of your buds and dramatically increase the lifespan of your gram.

First, only grind the marijuana right before use if possible—just as you're supposed to do with whole coffee beans in the morning. Of course in some cases, you have to pack it to go. If you plan on using it within a day or so and won't be able to grind on the go, it's best to pre-grind and take it in a small container. This way it's ready to roll or quickly pack any size bowl. It's also important to note that *you should always grind right before rolling a joint.* You don't want to grind too fine so that it ends up like dust, but packing with just the buds with stems is what leads to clogged, or "canoeing" joints. This can really ruin a smoke session and waste a lot of herb. If you're going to be using the ground up marijuana right away, it's best to just empty it out onto a business card—if not your own special marijuana card. A screen is preferable in all instances that it can be used. *(Note: Be sure to burn the screen at least once over before use to burn off any additional residue. As the screen changes color, you'll see it burn right off).*

After the marijuana is ground up on the card and the screen is in place, simply slide the desired amount from the card into the bowl or rolling paper/blunt. You'll notice that the bud grinds into a greater volume than it originally appeared in compact bud form, so it's common to have some left over. Just have a small container handy to keep what you haven't used . By using a screen, you also reduce the amount of still usable marijuana from being prematurely sucked through the fairly large holes found in the bottom of bowls and bongs.

It's best to roll joints/blunts/spliffs with a filter. This filter isn't actually meant to filter the potency of the marijuana like a cigarette filter, but simply to keep marijuana from entering the mouths of fellow tokers and from clogging the end with excess saliva and lip pressure build-up. Ultimately, this leads to not getting much out of your joint and a very unsatisfied toker.

• **Joints vs. Bowls:** Is it better to smoke joints or pack bowls generally? It's an age-old debate. Here's a little logic to ponder in helping you decide what is best for the situation. Unless you are getting fresh greens every time, most likely that dark pit of ash in the base of the bowl that you continue to milk for every ounce of smoke, has most likely already been stripped of its potency. If you've been the only one smoking the whole bowl, it may not really matter, although it's still not recommended. However, if you're on the receiving end of this bowl—which in large groups most of us are—it's a very watered-down experience. If on the other hand, we are passing around a joint or blunt, every hit an individual takes should technically be burning new bud. You'll provide the freshest, most potent, and enjoyable experience for others involved no matter how long it takes to get to them. Think about this concept the next time you're cashing that bowl after all your friends.

- **Loyal to the End:** One of the easiest habits to fall into when you're first exploring marijuana strains is to hold on to dear life to "the One" strain that you find and believe is perfect for you. Please consider that there are most likely many genetic variations of the "perfect" strain you like so much. As we learned already, tolerance is a factor. While your marijuana tolerance can be reset dramatically easier and faster than say alcohol, it can limit your experience and maximum effect experienced. It's great to find a strain that you love, but regard it as a guide stone in finding more strains that you will love. Ultimately, you'll build your arsenal to include your perfect strains for the perfect times of day and scenarios throughout your life. It's about finding the perfect healthy balance in your marijuana lifestyle. Exploring other options also allows you to share and introduce new strains to fellow tokers. After all, helping other marijuana users lead a more productive life is better for all parties involved.

- **Never Judge a Strain by Its Cover or Its THC Levels:** Remember that super purple amazing strain that lit up your eyes as soon as you saw it? It was a "must-have" bud you couldn't wait to show off to all your friends only to be left wanting after finally taking that first massive hit. Now you're pissed off and out some good money. Worst of all, you still need to get some decent marijuana. Feeling cheated? Well, there's truth on both sides here. As we now know, not all strains affect everyone the same way, so it's entirely possible that this strain just wasn't for you. That's why it's good to know what types of strains are generally effective for you and then branch out from there. You should be aware of other variables taking place that can contribute to a failed smoke session, other than the strain itself just not being "right" for you.

- **Bogus or Corrupted Labs:** There are a few truly good marijuana labs out there that provide accurate screenings and testing. Many others will inflate numbers to attract more business or because they can't afford to be on the cutting edge of the kind of technology needed to compete with finding accurate strain measurements. It can be incredibly expensive to keep up with the scientific discoveries being made with marijuana every day. Basically, this research continues to lead to inflated THC levels throughout the marijuana market. Bottom line: Depending on the individual, high THC /CBD levels may not be the most effective or the *most desirable for the person.* You may find that a mid-shelf or bottom-shelf strain (so long as it is clean) can deliver better or more desirable effects than a top-shelf, more expensive strain. Your strain journey isn't a competition with others, but a self-exploration of what is right for *you.* You may find you can live very happily on a mid-or bottom-shelf product, getting more beneficial effects, for a more modest budget over time.

• **Poor Curing by Grower:** This typically can lead to lots of crystals with little punch. This happens too often when beautiful buds don't deliver as anticipated. Sometimes Trichomes (THC crystals visible on the plant) can be like the push-up gel bra of the marijuana strain world. This letdown can be for a variety of reasons: If the head is gone, possibly so is a lot of the potency. Often the problem can be traced directly back to a mishap with the grower, usually during the curing process. One way to help to avoid these kinds of disappointments is *to use your nose as well.* Generally a well-done cure has great Trichome coverage as well as a very potent aroma. You should always take smell into account when searching for strains.

- **Poor Storage—Stale or Older Marijuana**: It's best to avoid all of these products. They can generally be spotted by their dry, flakey buds that have little to no smell left. Over time THC degrades the longer it's exposed to oxygen. While that doesn't always dramatically reduce the effects, it can play a role and should be a contributing factor in an educated consumer's purchase.

- **The Same Strains Are not Created Equal:** So you've been wanting for a long time to smoke that Skywalker OG you have heard a lot about. When you get some, it's not quite as "crystal-like" as you'd hoped and the smell isn't that much better than stuff you've been getting for years. Well, don't panic or be too disappointed, because this may not mean Skywalker OG isn't as great as you had hoped or heard; it's more likely that you either (1) found a poorly grown and cured batch of it being sold at a lower price; or (2) chose a mystery strain that had been renamed to be sold at a faster rate. It's important that you make sure you have a genuine sample, with ample Trichome coverage and a pungent smell before casting official judgment on any one strain.

- **Knowing Thyself Is the Key to Eternal Strain Happiness:** The best way to achieve this is to start a strain journal. Have your own rating system (maybe 1-5) and use stars for the ones that give you special desired effects (i.e.; pain or menstruation relief, sleep, anxiety relief, creativity, etc.). Navigating the strain world can be daunting even with a great database to choose from. One reliable outside source, marijuana.net, is an excellent reference site on the Internet.

It's easy to forget exactly what a strain was called and how it made you feel when switching so many strains over the course of the week, month or year. By simply creating your own rudimentary system, you'll be able to extrapolate your own strain likes, dislikes, and preferences, which will make you not only a more educated consumer, but ultimately, one step closer to creating your perfect balance with marijuana.

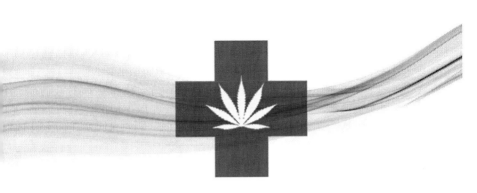

CHAPTER 4

GOING OUT INTO THE WORLD!

Now that we've built a strong foundation based on the important information offered in the earlier chapters, you're well on your way to becoming a modern-day, walking, talking beacon of light for other marijuana users everywhere. The remaining chapters of this book will focus mainly on how to apply many of these concepts to everyday scenarios. These tips will help you to use proper etiquette that will make your relationship with marijuana and the modern marijuana lifestyle a healthier and more informed one. Your goal is to be the ultimate well-rounded guest or host. It's time to get you out into the world!

First, there are a few things to keep in mind when encountering some everyday scenarios that should help empower you. If you follow the guidelines and advice below, you'll continue to build a more positive image for marijuana and avoid the "slacker stoner" label.

Being a Good Guest

It's important to understand that it's your responsibility to educate and share your knowledge of marijuana with fellow friends and family. Often the best way to share all you know is to lead by example.

Arrive on Time, But Not Early!

No one likes to be left waiting, and basically it's just rude. Whether you're going to meet a close friend or attending a business meeting, whether you've been smoking marijuana or not, you should always strive to be on time. It's a sign of mutual respect and shows your host that you value their time. If you're running late, it's courteous to let the host know. This will only reflect positively on you. Pothead flakes are notorious for showing up very late or sometimes, not at all. It also sets a good precedence for other events in your life. One way to make yourself stand out in today's world and not let marijuana sabotage your image is by simply being *someone of your word*. That one quality is a rarity, and big decision makers know it!! *Start with being where you say you will be, when you say you will be.*

Many times the host may be waiting for the entire group before beginning. There's a proper etiquette to follow when having a session. You really don't want to be so late as to—

- *Miss out completely.*
- *Be that "lame guest" who keeps your fellow tokers from getting started.*

On the other hand, arriving too early may throw the host off. As many stoners already know, we all have certain ways we like to prepare for things. You should expect the same of your host as well. Show some consideration and respect their prep time leading up to the event!

Bring Some Herb or Edibles!

While these are usually the best items to bring to a session for a variety of reasons, you must know your marijuana or edibles before you begin sharing. Only bring a strain relevant to the session and tolerance of fellow tokers. Bringing the wrong strain for the time and place can ruin the occasion. Having the marijuana pre-ground in a container is preferable so the host can add/use it in any way he/she desires. If you're bringing a pre-rolled joint or blunt, be sure to remember what you've learned about the proper rolling etiquette in order to provide the most pleasant, smooth experience possible for your fellow tokers.

If you're bringing edibles:
- *Bring enough for everyone to at least sample.*
- *Know the strength and dosage information.*
- *Give fair warning to everyone!!*

You want to make the session as pleasant as possible for everyone involved, which includes not overdoing it and making others uncomfortably high.

Don't Come Empty Handed!

As a guest, you should always bring something to the table: *No one* wants to be "the guy on the couch" or hang with him. Why?

Because *no one* wants to be pegged as a "moocher" or to have them around. I understand not everyone is rolling in dough, especially in this economy, so bringing enough Mary Jane for everyone all the time is usually not an option.

If you're not going to bring your own bud to the session—either because you can't afford to or just don't have access, here are some tips to help you validate your place in the session and contribute positively to the group:

- **Offer to Throw in Some Money**. Whether you're buying street marijuana, medical grade marijuana, or legal recreational marijuana, it all still costs money and can get expensive for the average person to smoke everyone up on a regular basis. While knowing growers and marijuana business owners has a few advantages, the average person usually doesn't have someone like that in their circle of friends. If you're unable to bring some bud to the table, it's often expected and considered courteous that you offer to throw in a fair amount of cash to help cover the amount used for the occasion—*insist when necessary!*

- **Pack Some of Your Friend's Favorite Party Snacks or Drinks**. A simple gift like a bag of snacks (but be mindful of any dieting going on) shows you've given thought to your fellow tokers and that you looked forward to the sessions. People really notice these kinds of small gestures.

- **Bring or Create a Fun Game or Movie to Watch.** Marijuana always goes well with games, especially in groups (avoid single player games). Playing games while using marijuana with friends is a popular pastime. Whether it's playing a board game, or the latest and greatest video game, or listening to old records, it keeps everyone engaged and active and having a good time. If money is an issue, this can bring a lot of fun to a group and make you a positive contributor and bringer of the fun. If bringing a movie, it's best to bring a cerebral yet exciting film; Sci-fi is always a good bet, but as usual, try to know your audience, so your choice is a big success.

- **No Money? No Games? No Herb?** So it's been just the worst year or years and you have nothing but the clothes on your back (and they're borrowed), you're really struggling to make a living, maybe crashing from couch to couch. Well, even in desperate times you should always avoid being a *"Moocher"* and when possible, *always contribute.* At the very least, a guest should arrive armed with interesting topics of conversation. You can always introduce an intellectual, philosophical and/or theological debate to help exercise the minds of yourself and your fellow smokers. As a bonus, being an engaging and informed conversationalist never fails to impress the fairer sex. Not that deep? In a pinch, learn something additional about marijuana to share, or just bring this book!

- **Don't Peer Pressure Your Friends.** We touched on this concept in earlier chapters. Peer pressure is generally an unpleasant experience, and you always want to provide the most enjoyable marijuana experience for others. Be respectful of others' tolerances and when someone wants to pass and has had enough, be respectful and oblige them.

- **Never Brag about Your High Tolerance.** While you might smoke more than anyone you know and feel proud of it, you aren't going to make anyone feel better by trying to make them feel inferior when it has absolutely no relevance. Most likely you're going to get a negative image for smoking more than anyone else they know. While these judgments may not be fair, you must make your best effort to avoid them.

- **Don't Blow Smoke in the Faces of Your Fellow Smokers.** Unless you've been specifically asked to do so, this is generally considered to be very rude, especially if you're smoking while someone is eating. However, often in the marijuana world it's common for someone to ask for a "shottie" or just for someone to pass second hand smoke on to him or her by blowing it in his or her direction. Sometimes the hit can be too harsh for new smokers. In these instances, blowing smoke directly at someone is considered to be okay but otherwise it would be deemed rude. For the most part, smoking marijuana while someone is eating isn't considered to be as rude as smoking a cigarette, but you should be aware of your surroundings and know the proper time and place for use. Always ask for permission from your host before you light up in their home. *Never assume burning marijuana indoors is okay. Always ask first.*

- **Look Out for New Marijuana Users.** Never revel in getting a new marijuana user too high. If done properly, introducing someone to marijuana is a privilege. It can open their entire life up in a healthy new direction. If you meet someone new to smoking marijuana, speak to them intelligently on the subject. Good information is hard to find and you can really help someone out by clearing up some common misconceptions or even the blatant false propaganda that they may not know is complete BS.

- **Don't Prejudge Others and be Open to Everyone.** As a guest, you should be open and respect-

ful of all of the other guests of the host. The marijuana demographic is not reserved to just the
young and cool, it reaches demographics larger
than 18-65, in all shapes, sizes, colors and creeds.
We're all connected and unity is not limited by
age, race and sex. It's to your advantage to culti-
vate relationships with all walks of life. It's only
then that we can really learn new things from
others. Marijuana is a glue that binds many of us
from all walks of life and it should be utilized as
a powerful networking tool.

• **Don't Be a "Dooby-Downer."** While it's good to
lean on friends for support, you should never
burden others with personal problems and/or
be the one known for whining about your life all
the time. There's a time and a place for this that
utilizes those friendships properly. If you're unhappy with your life, the key to change is *action*.
Constantly bitching and complaining and worry-
ing will get you nowhere and will probably just
annoy the hell out of those around you. If you
find that your friends and family have stopped
asking you how you are in general, *you're probably
one of those people.* If you must complain or rant
about something, or some injustice, at least have
a solution to follow it up; otherwise you're just
contributing to the noise. Remember: you always

want to make the experience the most pleasant for everyone and be a positive contributor, even in the face of distasteful subjects. No one wants to just hear all of your woes.

- **Don't Raid the Cabinets for Food!** Food, just like marijuana, is expensive. Although a host is generally responsible for supplying these items, a considerate and tactful guest knows he/she shouldn't expect them. Being invited over doesn't give you an entitlement to raid your host's cabinets and refrigerator for food. You never know what little thing was being saved and or how hard food may be to come by for your friend. If nothing is going to be being offered and you can't afford enough for everyone, bring your own favorite form of hydration and perhaps a personal snack. A good way to avoid these situations is to agree on food and beverages beforehand. Order out and split the tab or just eat ahead of time. Bottom line: you never want to be "that obnoxious guest" who just comes over, blazes, eats all the food, then passes out or leaves.

- **Know Your Limit.** Getting "tore up" or comatose on the couch at home may just be what you choose to do in privacy, but most people don't want to invite someone over to be a useless vegetable on their couch. Avoid this by not only choosing your strains wisely, as we have learned, but by also not over-indulging or caving to peer pressure. True friends should always be respectful of your boundaries and not try to push you outside of them for their own enjoyment or entertainment. If you begin to feel like you are getting a little "too" nice, kindly pass. This does not mean you are a "wimp" because you require less to get to that sweet spot. This is ultimately better for you because you require less and do not need large amounts or more expensive types of bud to get to your desired effect. By overindulging, you increase your tolerance unnecessarily, which will eventually require you to spend more money on herb both in the short and long term to keep up a tolerance you didn't need to raise so fast. Even if only for a short while, keeping your tolerance low as well as diversifying your strains is the most cost effective way to enjoy marijuana.

People rarely complain when another person passes because it allows more to go around for those of us who need it! Being a hog is bad for you in the long run, not only from a financial standpoint, but also in effecting the enjoyment of the plant in general. Plus, you're being annoyingly selfish amongst fellow tokers—and people will remember that.

- **A Warning!** Many marijuana users report that their first time smoking after using small to heavy amounts of alcohol can result in extreme nausea. If you're unfamiliar with how mixing alcohol and marijuana affects you, it may be best to try it on your own time first. Getting sick and ruining the occasion because you don't know your own limits even amongst friends is *not* an option. While true friends would still have your back, you never want to be a burden and put your friends in that position in the first place. In some cases, those who know they would be drinking ahead of time found that smoking marijuana before drinking can help eliminate the undesirable effects later on if smoking again after alcohol intake.

- **Don't Pass Out at Your Friends or the Event!** Stay engaged or take off. You never want to be a burden on your fellow tokers and furthermore, never want to inconvenience them or ruin their experience. If you're feeling tired, the proper thing to do is to excuse yourself early, and just go home and get some rest. You need to know your tolerance in order to avoid these situations in the first place. Again, even a small dose of prevention can go along way. If you're known to be prone to this type of smoking crash, maybe changing up strains, bringing your favorite pick-me-up drink, or cutting back on your intake can prevent this situation from happening. But if it's already too late because you've smoked too much, brought the wrong strain, or had too much of an edible, kindly apologize and ask your host for a place to rest until you feel okay enough to go home. The best advice of course, is to try to avoid being in these situations in the first place; however, sometimes they're unavoidable.

Remember: Any uncomfortable effects of marijuana that you may experience are always temporary, and the best thing for coming back down to "normal" is time. Keep in mind:

For the Ladies: Always be wary of situations where you may find yourself uncomfortably high or passed out in a stranger's or new friend's home. At all costs, always bring the number of a trusted cab company or maybe you should either save that *first* toke for when you're with your trusted friends, or experiment solo.

For the Gentlemen: We know how being the first to pass out at a party can follow you around for a lifetime. Better to not allow yourself to become a living canvas for your buddies to express themselves, especially in the digital age. Idle hands and unconscious friends are never a good combo!

- **Depart Safely**. While the jury is still out on the effect of marijuana on drivers, you know yourself better than anyone—never endanger the wellbeing of others or yourself. *If you feel out of sorts, don't risk it!* There are lots of unfortunate problems that you can incur when smoking and driving regardless of how "much better" of a driver you may be under the influence. The government wants money and while they can enforce laws and collect, they will. You may be a better, more cautious driver when you're high, but beware—it makes you an easier target for police to wring money out of through tickets and fines. Unfair? Yes it is, but understanding the game helps you play it smarter and helps you to avoid any unnecessary speed bumps in a world that already seems stacked against us.

Now that you're trained as an enlightened guest and you have some positive social smoking experience under your belt, you may feel inclined to host a special marijuana related get-together of your own. Building on everything I have outlined in this book to this point, you're now ready to become a perfect 420 host.

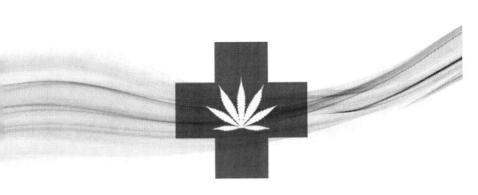

CHAPTER 5

ENTERTAINING AND THE MARIJUANA LIFESTYLE

Many factors should be taken into consideration when attempting to host your own marijuana themed get-to-gether. Marijuana can create many different effects amongst your guests and the best way to be an excellent 420 host, is to make sure they are as comfortable as possible. Since the marijuana culture is slightly different than your typical get-togethers, there are few things to keep in mind so that your epic "MJ Meet-up" doesn't turn into a stoner disaster.

Know Your Meds: For Your Guest's Sake and Your Own!
We've already explored the importance of knowing your meds and the effects of the individual strains in Chapter 3: *Know Your Meds*. It's not only very important to know for yourself, but for properly executing a party when most likely you will

be supplying the bud. If you plan on having a chill barbeque on the beach all day filled with fun in the sun and activities galore, you better be packing a sativa or hybrid in general to make sure your group isn't too baked to participate. That goes for stimulating conversation as well. However, for a more seasoned group, anything may go. You must always be aware of your guests and try your best to accommodate their individual tolerances and strain preferences if and when possible.

Know Your Crowd

By simply paying attention to your friends, you can soon understand your guests and their marijuana preferences. That way, you can really provide the ultimate blazing environment whether in a large group or just with your favorite blazing buddy.

Set the Table for Success and to Impress

A modern 420 host expresses his appreciation for his guests by making them as comfortable as possible. This relates directly to knowing your crowd. While choosing the right strains for the occasion is first and foremost, the supplemental items to make your party as enjoyable as possible should be your next priority. Preparation is key. Because you know your friends well, you can find out their favorite types of snacks and preferred blazing beverage by paying attention to a few of your previous smoke sessions together. It's totally worth it to go out of your way to provide your guests not *just* a snack and drink but *the perfect* snack or drink!

Maintain a Positive Atmosphere

Just like the most successful places of recreation such as bars, restaurants, and nightclubs that create the best vibe for the customers, you should also aim to create the best vibe for your guests given the resources at your disposal. A little music and lighting can go a long way here. Just be sure not to go crazy with candles that make it weird for your guests. There can also be an "adjustment" period for some people as they acclimate to the marijuana you're offering. Music can play a huge role here by filling in that potentially silent passage of time. Heavy metal music may not be the best choice in soothing your guests, but it really depends on the crowd. Try to appeal to the others with your music selection. If in doubt, you can always go with reggae music!

Provide the Entertainment

Whether you've planned a full-on gamer night, an epic movie marathon, an intense poker night, a hike, or Frisbee on the beach, always make sure you're prepared. Here a few scenarios to keep in mind depending on how you may plan to entertain.

For Gamers (Ladies Welcome)

Always make sure you have a game appropriate for the number of players present. It's really easy to isolate yourself or others from the fun if there are only so many controllers. Aim for multiplayer games and also try to keep the amount of players invited limited. You can also get online with others, possibly with another group. Generally, gaming is best for just you and your best gaming buddy because you can get into deeper game play and work a nice blazing routine in, but some sport games like golf make it fun for up to 4 people at once. Cool fighting or racing games (girls tend to be more likely to try them also) with quick turnovers are good and let a lot of guests get involved and take turns. No one wants to come over and see how awesome you are at your games all night no matter how cool you may think it is. Save it for online or that's all you may have left one day! Ladies, this can be a great way to meet new guys and or bond with your new hubby. Men generally hate talking on the phone, but they'll game with you all day or maybe even trade a gaming session for a yoga session? Imagine the possibilities!

The Movie Night

Have your movie selection ready to go, and make sure that it's an appropriate genre for your guests. Try and make it something that invokes thought or laughter. Have the herb, munchies, and drinks ready to go upon arrival. But be conscious of your guests' dieting needs.

Board Games and Activities/Sports

Okay, this will seem obvious, but make sure you have all the parts or equipment beforehand to any game you choose to play. Usually, the hardest thing to do is to get everyone together in the busy world. Once they are there, it really sucks when you don't have the equipment necessary to actually do the event you planned. Not only does this seem overly terrible after everyone is high, it'll reflect poorly on being "that guy" who organized the football game but forgot the football, or who hosts "movie night" but forgets to provide the movie. Sure that sounds funny, but how do you think it ultimately makes you look to others? Do yourself and your guests a favor and *always double check you have all the equipment before the actual event.* Our free time is valuable and sometimes pretty scarce. We should cherish and respect it. Do the little things to avoid being unprepared, no matter what the theme of the evening.

Provide Stimulating Topics of Conversation

It's good to challenge the minds of those around you by providing stimulating topics of conversation and introducing new concepts to others, sometimes challenging the inconsistencies and injustices they see in the world around them. Sometimes the right movie can really set the stage for great debate sessions if you can't find a way to bring up a specific topic. Perhaps you could consider George Orwell's classic book, *1984* as an interesting place to start during your next session with your friends. The fact that its most relevant days may still be ahead is a whole other problem we don't have the pages to cover.

Expect Your Guests to Be Unprepared

Sometimes we're truly busy and sometimes we just plain forget things. Due to the stigmas still associated with marijuana use, tokers are also usually forced outside or to become creative in choosing a place to toke up. Many times, these situations can lack traditional comfort and shielding from the elements. People can find themselves uncomfortably unprepared very quickly. You should come to expect this from your guests, prepare for the possibility and not hold it against them. Carrying little extras for the activity or weather can really help make the experience much more pleasant for someone who may just not have been prepared. For example: extra sunscreen, shades, extra hoodie or shorts for a summer party. Remember to keep everyone hydrated!

Lead by Example!

We covered how to use proper etiquette in joining or setting your own circle in Chapter 4: *Going Out in the World.* This is your chance to lead by example. Take the opportunity to teach and correct on your home turf so not to be rude when you're a guest somewhere else. It's a fine line between teaching and preaching and helping and being the damn know-it-all. You need to walk this line carefully and know the right time to interject and offer advice or when to just relax and let it go. In every case, the best thing to do is lead by example. If you do teach, go more for the concept and why it's a good thing for your fellow tokers to know, rather than just regurgitating information to sound smart.

When Possible—Provide the Healthiest Options for Your Guests

At the minimum, alert your guests to the alternatives— especially if a first time smoker is in your midst. As we have explained, smoking is still the most harmful way to use marijuana. Vaporizing, while expensive, and edibles, if dosed properly, are the safest, most potent ways of using marijuana. It's important to spread this knowledge to others. Many people's sole reason for not using it is because of the stigma attached to smoking, and although very deserved in regards to cigarettes, it still holds some truth in regards to marijuana smoke also. Thankfully, the vaporizer and edible market have largely evolved over the years to offer high tech ways to perfectly vaporize and consistently dose edibles, which offer zero known harmful side effects when combined with healthy ingredients. Keep in mind that vaporizing may seem like an expensive investment for you, but maybe not your new friend who is now convinced by you and has some extra money lying around to invest in his health. Now he has a volcano you both get to use, simply because you educated and looked out for him. Karma can be rewarding.

Treat Beginners with Special Care

Keeping in mind the concepts we learned from the earlier chapters, it's imperative to always introduce a new marijuana smoker properly. Be very delicate and bring them on at their own pace. This is a privilege and how you introduce this plant to someone for the first time can have very positive or negative long-term effects for the person. It is not to be taken lightly and should be treated with the utmost care and respect. Consider it as being responsible for "birthing" a new stoner into the world. Newbies need to have the best chance at success and balancing their marijuana lifestyle so that it's only a positive force in their life. You not only want this for your fellow toker but long term, it's for the good of all marijuana users. They say change for the future starts with our children; same concept here.

Be Extremely Careful with Providing Guests with Edibles!

This can prove to be very challenging and you need to pay close attention. First, you must try and find consistently dosed edibles. If your guests are inexperienced with edibles, it's very important to give them this friendly advice:

1. *Start with a small amount first, depending on the overall dose of the edible.* Wait around 25-40 minutes then add a little more if they want to increase the effect. You can always add a little more; you don't want to be in the position where you regret eating too much!

2. *Try and find edibles that are already scored in single doses.* Many chocolate bars have this convenience making them better for sharing in groups, rather than using a cookie or brownie that tends to crumble more often than not, making it harder to dose effectively. It's also common for potency to gather around the edges of brownie trays, leaving them inconsistent throughout. This happens with cookies sometimes as well.

3. *The size and strength of a person has nothing to do with how the plant will affect them.* Even the mightiest can fall to the smallest of potent edibles. In fact, since the active components of marijuana are actually fat soluble, a heavier body weight usually leads to an extended effect on the user.

4. *Eating on an empty stomach can expedite the effect of the edible;* while on the other hand, eating an edible on

a full stomach may make the edible take longer to find its way into your digestive track, thus delaying the effects of the edible for the user.

5. *Eating additional food after the edible has taken effect has been known to extend the effect on the user.* This is largely due to more of the THC and/or CBD being absorbed through your small intestine. By eating additional food, you're pushing the edible further into your small intestine where nutrients from food are more effectively absorbed.

6. *Sometimes an edible can be the gift that keeps on giving.* Unlike smoking marijuana, eating marijuana does not provide the user with instant effects, and in some cases after it does finally kick in, can come in unpredictable waves for the user. Just when you think it's worn off, you can be hit with another wave. This can also be true of still feeling the effects of edibles the day after taking them. It's not uncommon for someone who eats a high potency edible late at night to continue to feel that buzz the next morning when they wake up.

7. *Marijuana drinks are known to have slightly different effects than edibles.* Generally, they can begin working much faster and can provide varied effects on the individual that are sometimes slightly different than smoking or eating. Cannabis condiments or marijuana sauces such as BBQ sauce, ketchup, mustard etc. may also have this type of effect on the user.

8. *Always let your guests know that nobody has ever died or overdosed from any form of marijuana use.* A lot of people freak out and rush to the hospital only to feel very silly afterwards. Just knowing this information beforehand can go a long way in preventing a total freak-out by a new user. The "bad trip" usually comes from inside their head, along with insecurities fueled by the inexperience of using marijuana for the first time.

9. *Beware of homemade edibles.* Proper dosing has become a science and unless your host has taken some serious steps in knowing what they are doing or *you* have a very high tolerance, I would avoid trying "random" edibles from people. Although, learning the proper recipes and techniques can help provide an amazing experience as well as potentially opening up a new career path if at the right time and place.

Always try to make your fellow toker's experience as pleasant as possible. Providing knowledge can be equally or more important than providing the actual marijuana, especially when it comes to introducing edibles to others (Warning: you may lose your audience without the marijuana).

As we move on from edibles, there are a few more important things to remember when hosting a marijuana-themed get together:

- **Be Prepared for Crashers.** While most people understand that an invitation to hang out usually isn't an invitation to crash on the couch, it's more than likely if you are having a marijuana themed get-together you may have someone that inhaled a little more than they could handle and needs to sleep it off, or more likely has already been crashed out for the last half of the party and now you can't wake them up. There's usually going to be a little collateral damage from over-indulgence, so it's a good idea to at least have sleeping materials prepared for your guest if a bed or couch is not available. A pillow and blanket can and should be provided at the minimum, so that your guests will be as comfortable as possible. If you are not prepared to be kind in these situations, then maybe being a guest is better suited for you than hosting.

- **Never Shun or Exploit Your Guest's Insecurities for a Laugh.** This rule is pretty self-explanatory and is one of the core concepts understood by the modern day, intelligent, well-informed, and compassionate marijuana user.

The choice of themes for your marijuana parties may be endless, but always remember that no matter where the theme may take you and your guests, making the experience as pleasant and enjoyable for those around you should always be a priority. Be happy to do it!

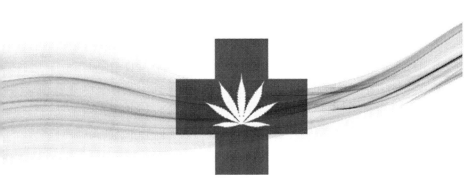

CHAPTER 6

FRIENDS AND FAMILY AND
THE MODERN TOKER

We discussed some tips for being the ultimate host or guest in the previous chapters. Generally, within the marijuana culture, we do hang out a lot either hosting friends or being hosted by others. While this is largely due to marijuana use not being tolerated in public areas, "the times, they are a changin'." Laws are easing up and tokers everywhere are braving the world with a new sense of confidence, especially in groups.

The bad news is that there are times when the "bad apples" are at their worst, seemingly determined to ruin it for the rest of us. In these group or social settings, you and your friends should avoid creating a bad image for not only yourself but for the everyday marijuana user as well. Here are some tips to avoid being dubbed the "Cheech" or "Chong" stoner of your group and to help in not letting your love of marijuana get in the way of you or the friends around you who may not smoke.

Not everyone will see marijuana the way you do, no matter how reasonably the logic is presented. If you choose to bring your marijuana use out into public, it's important that you don't fuel the stereotypes that unfairly keep others from realizing the great benefits of this plant while simultaneously respecting the rights and opinions of others.

Socializing With Friends

- **Always work harder to keep your word.** Flakes are a dime a dozen and only keep real progress from being made.
- **Always brings enough to share.** You know how many buddies will be there and if you're planning on bringing your own marijuana, have enough to share.
- **Know your marijuana, especially what it brings into the lungs.** Knowing the type of marijuana you're smoking is not only good for you, but you should always be able to communicate to others what type of strain they are smoking, what type of effects the group should expect, and you should be sensitive to the tolerance of others. You should never intentionally try to make your fellow tokers uncomfortable or have a poor marijuana experience. Many people are unaware of the multiple types of strains and all the different

benefits available from trying different types of marijuana. Always try to match the right strain with the right activity. If you're so informed, pass this knowledge on to others to help create a better experience for them. Sometimes, explaining the "why" can make all the difference—not just for that day, but possibly for a lifetime. If you are new to the scene, it's important to ask questions and become a more informed marijuana user.

- **Always conceal smell and grass discreetly.** You never want to draw unnecessary attention to you or your group—whether you're all marijuana users or not; but this is especially true if you're with some friends who just don't use it. You also don't want to run the risk of it being sniffed out by someone nearby (or by police, depending on what state you are in).

- **Never risk the fun of the group to get high unless everyone else is in agreement.** No one wants to get thrown out of "the big game" you've all been waiting to go to all year because you just couldn't wait to toke or fit it in beforehand. It makes you look like a weak addict and pisses off your friends who may not enjoy marijuana to the extent you do. In today's world, the edible options are mounting and so is the quality; therefore, those types of scenarios should be dwindling as time goes on.

- **Don't get thrown out of the bar for lighting up.** Because you just *had* to smoke and their "rules" are stupid. We are already extremely lucky in our lifetime to have access to marijuana the way we do. Yes, there's a long way to go, but rules are there for a reason, and if you break them, there will be consequences. One consequence will likely be your friends will invite you out with them less. It's also important to remember that no matter what the state law allows, if push comes to shove anywhere in the US, federal law would prevail and you could be brought up on marijuana charges.

- **Don't ruin the evening if you don't have any marijuana.** Try not to put yourself in those situations and when you find yourself there, don't blame others or take it out on them. It makes you look weak and addicted and that may concern friends or family and draw unwanted attention and unfortunate speculation to your marijuana use. Again, a dose of prevention can really go a long way here.

- **Don't be the "bitchy caffeine drinker."** We all know somebody who announces, "If I don't get my coffee in the morning, I'm a real asshole to be around." Guess what? Most likely they're really just an asshole, coffee just helps hide it. It's the same concept here: Not having your Mary

J doesn't give you an excuse to be a frustrated brat! If you feel it does, you should be more focused on solving why you're being an ass in the first place. Don't let this be you!

• **Be respectful.** Be mindful of how significant people in your family and friends' lives see you because unfortunately, early on and as we get older, they end up carrying a lot of influence over the people we hang out with. This goes for parents, girlfriends, boyfriends, wives, husbands or children. Try to present yourself as the kind of person they would want their significant people to be around. After you've established the right impression, go ahead and be yourself with your pal.

• **Don't "pot-block" your single friends.** Too often, just as the night begins to heat up at the after-party, someone has to pass the grass around. For the most part, this is *never* a bad thing, but in certain scenarios, smoking up the crowd may hurt your *ultimate* plans, as sometimes combinations of grass and alcohol can be disastrous. Depending on the strain, the effects can be less predictable on the user than your friends may had hoped and lead to an early and very disappointing departure by your guests.

Tipping the Scales in Your Favor

Here are a few little tips and concepts to contemplate when

reaching for that check at the end of the night or just in general. It's just classy if you can afford to tip well—even a server who has prejudged you. Not only is it more in the spirit of marijuana use, tipping well gives us all a good name. If you insist on looking like the typical stoner, at least make us look good by being a good tipper. After all, it's our fellow man struggling to survive in this economy just as we do—and it's good Karma.

You and your friends may not get chased out of your favorite hangout, whether it be a diner or restaurant, if you throw them a tip *based on the amount of time you hang, not the amount you order*. In the end, they just want to wait on tables with higher checks because they're more likely to get a larger tip. Waiting on you and your friends who are high and ordering a few coffees over the course of two hours can understandably be quite infuriating when the server's tip is only a small percentage of a few nonalcoholic drinks. However if you can scrape together enough cash between you and your friends to leave a decent tip, what you order will be irrelevant to the server in most cases and they will tolerate your limited ordering on the menu in the future. The server gets as good a tip as they would for busting their ass working tables for three complaining families, just to let you and your friends hang all night hassle free filling up on a few drinks. Just consider it your price to hang and not be bothered. Everyone wins! If stoners were known to be notoriously good tippers, your hoodie might get you better service!

Remember: Never let your use of marijuana isolate you

from your friends or knowingly let it get in the way of having a positive experience with those you care about in your life. In the next chapter, we'll cover how to navigate some more common everyday scenarios to help you avoid being stereotyped, unfairly judged or looked down upon in real world settings.

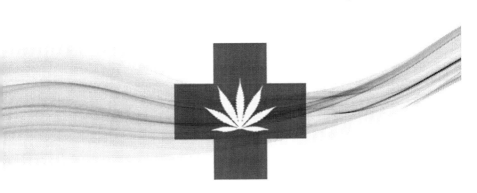

CHAPTER 7

THE MODERN MARIJUANA USER'S
DAILY GUIDE

Now that I've given you a crash course in etiquette and how to handle yourself around friends and family to ensure you don't make yourself look bad or make them feel uncomfortable, we can start to curb some of your everyday habits. It's very important not to let yourself fall into the stigmas and stereotypes commonly associated with marijuana and do your part to help lift them going forward.

Starting the Day

Before we get too much into the specifics, let's introduce the concept of "waking and baking." It *can* be awesome, if you know your strains well enough. No matter what you plan to accomplish over the course of the day, if you don't know what type of strain you're packing, you're rolling the dice as to wheth-

er or not you're going to maintain the same motivation for
your project after finishing your toke. The strain you choose
for your daily "wake and bake" may set the pace for the rest of
the day and is not to be decided lightly. Just as breakfast is the
most important meal of the day, the strain you start with can
have a lot of influence on the way your day goes. Many smoking "ruts" get started from people unknowingly using heavier,
more lethargic, even sleepy strains early in the day for longer
periods of time. Unfortunately, in a lot of cases, people don't
have many options available and are typically limited to scarce
diversity. Often they are unable to tell what effects they will
have at all from the strain. Here are a few common everyday
scenarios that you should be conscious of as you move through
your day.

Part 1
Ordering in Line

All too often the task of ordering in public while "high" has
intimidated the marijuana user, sometimes to a point where
it makes that desired goal seem unattainable. In this section
I want to talk about how using everything you've learned thus
far, you can be cool and confident while mingling amongst the
rest of the world all while remaining under the influence of
your favorite "companion."

  If you've learned and put into use the information and tips
from earlier chapters in regards to etiquette, articulation, and
things to avoid, then keeping in mind some of the following

may help to make your public encounters go from intimidating to ordinary.

Consider a few concepts first...

- Most of the people you encounter when you're going out tend to be strangers that have never met you before. They don't know the difference between what you're like "normal" or "high." If you take some of the precautions we mentioned earlier such as Visine, washing, etc., you can avoid any other red flags signaling that you are stoned. The rest is all in how you carry yourself. Obviously if you start cracking up uncontrollably for no apparent reason, it may raise an eyebrow or two. In that case, it may just be best to wait until you come down to a more manageable high before you start gallivanting around town. Otherwise, making eye contact and watching your articulation can really help keep you under the radar.

- Being stoned shouldn't ever be something to be ashamed of in the first place, especially if you can speak intelligently on the subject so as to put any doubters to shame. Being discreet is usually the best course of action but you should always prepare to defend your actions proudly.

Here are some ideas to consider so that you don't stand out or get yourself in uncomfortable "high" situations when ordering in, on the phone, or in line:

1. **Know what you want beforehand.** This can really make all the difference! There's usually a pretty large menu for everyone to see while they wait. If you're the first one in line and know you're going to take a minute, step aside and let everyone go until you know what you want. Your one "high minute" is probably more likely five "normal minutes" to everyone else and a line with angry people can form behind you. Before you get all mad at *them* for "rushing" *you* take a minute to realize that not everyone may have the luxury to be able to enjoy marijuana as freely and as often as you may be able to. You may be the one in a rush one day and the last thing you'll need is some spaced out, indecisive "stoner" holding you up for a half hour just to get a cup of coffee, when in the end, the stoner just ended up ordering a simple coffee but "couldn't decide" with *all* the options. Don't be that person. Know what you want beforehand.

2. **Don't reek of marijuana in public.** Until enough of us become the change we want to see out there, we will be exposed to constant criticism and subject to unfair stigmas and stereotypes whenever we associate ourselves with marijuana. If you haven't masked your smell and they suspect you're stoned, you're opening up yourself for judgment. I'm not saying it's right, but if you want to fly under the radar, it's better to take all

precautions. Stinking like skunk paints a major bull's-eye on you and draws unnecessary attention to you and whomever you may be with.

3. **Use Visine and make eye contact.** Unless you've built up a solid tolerance to getting red-eye it's always good to keep a little Visine or some kind of red-eye relief handy. A lot of times it's better to put in a few drops before you actually blaze if possible, then use a few drops again right after you're done, if necessary. Always having Visine around is not only good for you, but could bail out a fellow toker in a variety of emergency scenarios. If you and your buddy's eyes look blunted, it puts you on the radar. Sunglasses are an option depending on if you are outdoors, but generally, keeping the shades on at night or indoors is also somewhat suspect because that telegraphs that you are under the influence but leaves it up to the imagination of the person judging you (which most likely will be worse than the actual truth).

4. **Detach from your cell phone while you're giving your order.** I know this might be one of the most radical concepts we have introduced thus far, but bear with me. How does it feel when you are talking to someone and they're just looking down at their phone and not really paying attention? Generally, pretty crappy, right? Infuriating even? So why the hell do we do it? Cell phone etiquette has gotten out of control and

you must make a conscious effort not to fall victim to excessive cell phone use.

5. **Use good manners.** Manners can take you a long way and help to further make you distinctive in an otherwise seemingly saturated world. Start with greeting the person and making eye contact. Whether it's just, "Hi, how are you?" Or a quick "Good morning, good afternoon, or good evening", you're telling the other person that you recognize you are interacting with a human being and you respect that time, no matter how fleeting. "Please" and "thank you" go a long way and seem to be nearly lost in a world of growing misguided self-entitlement. Use it to your advantage to mold the dynamic of your engagements with others in a more positive way from beginning to end. "Thank you, have a good one…" That's not so hard is it? You can even try and mix it up to get creative, I assure you it won't hurt.

Part 2
Cell Phone Etiquette

Just how bad has this excessive cell phone use gotten in our culture? Let's try and put it in perspective: In today's world when most children are born, rather than seeing the faces of the doctor, mother or father, they get the newest versions of smart-phones released over the past few years staring at them. Yes, of course I exaggerate, but no wonder we establish such a relationship with our phones—it's practically one of the first things we see when we're born. Scary isn't it?

Unfortunately this relationship often can start right at birth with either the parental assisted "selfie" close-up shots as the baby comes out of the womb or a digital video ready to download to their Facebook page or some other social media site. The cell phone seems to be an attachment that follows kids through their childhood right into adulthood. Today's generation of kids seems most comfortable keeping a phone between them and others. The result is that cell phones are limiting the connections people can make between one another. There will always be time to check the Internet and social media pages to see what's going on in the world, but a responsible marijuana user should know what's happening in real time. The personal connection you make with others that involve using all of your senses is the best way to experience life.

A cell phone is only a tool to help assist you to make direct connections with others—not to replace them. Try to exercise self-control when using your cellphone. There are a number of good ways to avoid giving off a bad image of your lifestyle choices unintentionally.

These tips will help you to keep from letting your cell phone negatively affect your relationships with others:

1. **Avoid excessive use in front of others.** You don't want to be the annoying person who is *always* on the cell phone. Whether you are the girlfriend no one can ever have a "real" conversation with, the boyfriend who "never"

listens because you're *always* on your damn phone, or the parents whose child resents them because they're always on their phone talking business and don't care about their kid's life, people feel disrespected when you choose to use your phone excessively during a shared time together. It says to them that your phone is more interesting than everything they bring to the table as a human being. If that's how you feel, save them the frustration and don't make plans. If not, show some respect and get to know the person you're with. Forging real relationships with people can really make life's journey easier when times get tough as they usually do for everyone at some point. That being said, we have phones for a reason and sometimes things come up and you need to take a call or respond to an important email. That's fine, but you should always explain the necessity as best as you can and apologize to the person you're with. Most people will appreciate that you're recognizing the value of their time and you wouldn't knowingly put them in this situation if you had another choice.

2. **High dialing.** You're just sitting around smoking your favorite herb on your day off. You start thinking of all your old smoking buds or just have a day to make all those "catch-up" calls you owe? Before you dial up your buddies or favorite family members, make sure to keep in mind the following tips so you can

avoid drawing negative attention to yourself for your marijuana use:

- **Remember who you are calling.** We've all had a time or two when we can't remember who we're calling *while the phone is actually ringing.* This can sometimes be a short-term side effect of marijuana. Repeat the name of whomever you're calling three times to yourself in your head beforehand to remember. If you do happen to forget before they pick up, hang up right away. Don't stay on the line and wait for them to pick up and leave you sounding stupid trying and stumbling to figure out who you've got on the line. The person on the other end knows it's you—*you* called *them,* remember? It may be funny to you and even to them at the moment but if it's friends or family you haven't spoken with in a long time, they only have these conversations to refer to. While you might be kicking ass in all aspects of your daily life, they only know what they get from the limited impression of you that you share with them over the phone. If you call and immediately forget the name of the person you're calling, they'll probably laugh it off with you, but believe me, it'll only hurt yourself in the long run.

- **Know what you basically want to talk about before you call**. It's important not to call up your friend or family member—especially your mother—and constantly forget why you called or, because your concept of time can be different when you're high, drift into a long "high" pause on the other end.

- **Make a list.** A short note with a few bullet points of what you want to talk about can be an effective tool to use. This way, even if you do space out, you can come back on topic and/or be ready to start another one without missing a beat. This lessens the chance of making your friends or family question your marijuana use.

- **Avoid excessive coughing.** Vaporizing or edibles are the preferred method to avoid this altogether. If this isn't an option and you've developed a regular cough, it may seem like just background static to you, but hacking away can raise a major concern amongst your loved ones. As I have advised, you can avoid the cough by using safer methods of marijuana altogether. At least avoid the inevitable lecture you'll get by just keeping the coughing to a minimum while you're on the phone. Remember, even as you become more enlightened about the wonderful aspects of marijuana, most people still associate marijuana as taboo (legalized pot states included) so you must work harder not to fuel that fire that will leave you open to unjustified criticisms reinforced by the old stoner stereotypes of an earlier era.

3. **Keep a beverage handy.** Staying hydrated is also very important because cottonmouth can sneak up on you, so it's good to have some beverage for the throat readily available. You never know when a rant may come

and/or just a lengthy catch up conversation.

4. **Calling in sick or cancelling.** It's important to not tip off your marijuana use when calling in sick or leaving a message to cancel. Maybe you're really not feeling your business meeting after waking and baking that Indica. We all have those days. There's nothing wrong with rescheduling every now and then as long as you understand that the proper thing to do on these occasions is to give as much notice to the other person as possible. With friends, while you generally have more leeway, they should still feel respected. If you're calling into work, you have less room for error and it's imperative you don't tip off your marijuana smoking to the person on the line.

5. **Toke *after* the call as a reward.** If you just get too high and you have serious calls to make, it's better just to wait until after the calls are finished. Get the call out of the way as early as possible and then you can relax without the stress of messing up later while you're high and enjoying your last-minute day off. This is recommended for business or conference calls as well. Sometimes you only get one chance to make an impression, why take the risk when you can just wait a little while until after the business is done.

6. **Ordering food.** When the "munchies" kick in at the peak of the high, ordering food can sometimes be a

problem. If you're ordering with others, it's a smart move to try and get them to do it for you. If everyone is too high to call in an order, there are a few ways to help solve the problem.

- *Make a list with all the orders on it.* If you can keep from cracking up on the line, having a list makes this process much easier. Also make sure to have the delivery address and a callback number ready if you're not at home.

- *Offer to get the door instead.* If you have anxiety about calling in the order or simply don't want to, a fair trade-off is to be the one to answer the door and deal with the delivery when it comes in. By "get" I don't mean "pay" for it all (of course pay your share), but be the one to actually physically get up and do the talking and tipping (keep in mind what we already learned about tipping in Chapter 6). Remember, there's a good chance that you'll see the delivery guy again and he'll be handling your food in the near future. That's just a little food for thought when deciding whether or not to be a cheap-ass. On the other hand, if you're the type who dreads person-to-person contact, maybe offering to make the call to place the order may be more up your alley. The important thing is to help contribute and be willing to compromise for the good of the group—especially when it comes to a "munchies" situation.

7. **Avoid embarrassing photos or video.** Life is very long

and hopefully we challenge ourselves to change over time. In today's world, unlike any other generation before us, most people have the ability to document their lives via social media. You're creating a footprint that will live long after you do and it will stalk your public profile forever—for better or worse. Google will not go away. Just keep in mind that what you may think is so *cool* now, may hurt your odds with that great job, new love interest, or school application if they just decide to do a little Internet search on you. Odds are they will.

8. **Avoid being the *one* who takes compromising photos or video.** To expand on #7, *you must always respect the privacy of fellow stoners.* It's totally unacceptable to be the one making a smoking situation uncomfortable for others. When you're smoking marijuana with another person, a special bond is shared that usually allows people to let their guard down because they're comfortable with *you*, not because they want you to exploit how goofy they can be in a private session with their friends or family.

Part 3
Munchies & Grocery Shopping

A crucial part of any marijuana user's life is finding nourishment. This is an unavoidable task unless you always order in, eat out or are lucky to have your own personal chef. In many cases, we're forced to hit the grocery store. Like many other things, a toke can make even the most routine tasks seem more enjoyable, so if you must blaze before hitting the store, there are some things that you may want to consider so as to make the experience as smooth as possible:

1. **Make a list.** This can make all the difference. Knowing what you need and not letting yourself divert from your list is the best way to ensure a quick and effective shopping experience. Without a list, you're likely to end up with a million things you craved while you were at the store but forget the main item you came in for.

2. **Keep up with shopping.** Try not to limit your shopping to once a month when you need to pick up everything. This helps to keep your cart or basket light and the checkout time more efficient.

3. **Meet and greet the cashier.** Direct eye contact and a casual, "Hi! How are you?" is common courtesy when interacting with salespeople and cashiers.

4. **Pros and Cons of self-checkout.** Many times, being publicly "stoned" lessens your desire to interact with other people on any level. But when you try to use self-checkouts to make your life easier and discreet, the self checkout option ends up making everything a lot more complicated and may even draw more attention to you than had if you'd used the old fashioned way. There's a reason why stores have an attendant on duty on a regular basis. At times, it doesn't go smoothly. On the flip side, you don't have to be paranoid that the

cashier is judging you for all of your Hostess baked goods and cat food!

5. **Don't buy perishable items in bulk.** Once you're in the store, you'll be tempted by all of the delicious items on display. The "jones" to buy it and eat it all now can lead to a seriously overloaded cart of perishables. Be aware: expiration dates are not always your friend when you buy perishable items in bulk. Most times you can munch away indulgently over time with non-perishables. There's really no harm, but cash can be hard to come by in today's economy and you should be diligent not to be wasteful of either your funds or your food. After all, the more you save, the more you have available for Mary J! If you can't freeze something or don't have room in the fridge, make sure you can eat it that day or very soon. Having a fridge full of spoiled food doesn't reflect well on you. Plus, basically your hard-earned cash rots away right in front of you.

Grocery shopping should be very important in the average toker's daily life. What you stock on your shelves and make available for munchies can have a drastic effect on your health and energy in your life. Many people blame marijuana for weight gain. The truth is if you know your strains, you can avoid those types that cause munchies in general. There are many (usually Sativas) that don't have this effect, but not always. The best thing to do is not to *avoid* the munchies, but to *anticipate* them and prep with healthier foods you enjoy. I'm not saying that you shouldn't indulge every now and then, but if marijuana is a day-to-day companion, you can't *only* eat your favorite junk foods. That's a problem with self-control—not marijuana. It's important to pick up some healthy high munchies, so when you do get that uncontrollable hunger, you're filling your body with good vitamins and nutrients. So, replace that Hostess cupcake or bag of chips with some strawberries and light whipped cream. Switch out that Big Gulp soda for a bottle of water or iced tea. Balancing marijuana with good nutrition and some form of exercise is truly the key to living a healthy, balanced, positive marijuana lifestyle.

Part 4
Exercise

While common misconceptions usually make marijuana users out to be the more unproductive, lazier portion of the population, statistically, the opposite seems to have been proven true over the last few years. Not only has marijuana been linked to helping regulate insulin, marijuana smokers have been found to be leaner in general than the average person. It seems the marijuana and alcohol statistics have been lumped in with each other for convenient purposes of distorting the truth once again. While getting a gym membership and pumping up is usually the most common option available to people who want to get in shape, it's not right for a lot of people. Keep the following ideas in mind when bringing marijuana into your life on a daily basis.

Find a Way

The most important thing to remember is this: *It doesn't have to be at a gym to be considered a workout!* Anything that gets your blood pumping can be considered good exercise and is certainly better than doing nothing at all. If you hate gyms, find an outdoor activity you like. Anything as easy as walking, hiking, riding a bike or playing an activity with others either daily or once a week can really help alleviate stress and connect you with nature. If money is an issue, those activities are free of charge. If you hate the outdoors and live through video games and computers—well you should really work on that, but in the meantime, try doing just 20 push ups if your kill death ratio on Call of Duty is under 1.00 per death match, or every time you have to watch a commercial in between your favorite shows. That can really get you in shape fast and make commercials more tolerable if you don't have DVR. Maybe switch it up to sit-ups or lunges to work out other parts of your body. You'll be surprised: it can really add up over time. The concept here is that it's okay to not be a "gym" person, but it's not okay to boycott all exercise. Where there is a will, there is a way, so put some of that high creativity to use here. No one else is gonna do it for you—but *you.*

Stretching Is the Key to Longevity

We really have the popularity of yoga to thank for this. There are 70+ year old entertainers performing things that most people in their early 20's, with average exercise habits, can't do on their best day. Yoga is redefining what a person's retirement years can be in a positive way for those who make stretching a part of their life at earlier ages. As much as you'd like to believe they were taking magic beans, yoga is almost always the secret for finding the fountain of youth. If you've dismissed this form of exercise as a bunch of sunshine and butterfly nonsense, I challenge you to take a 90-minute Bikram class and still keep that opinion. People of any age can take up yoga, which can help increase vitality and core strength.

Stay Hydrated

This is something you already know to do on a regular basis when using marijuana, it's even more important when increasing your physical activity.

Keep It Clean

Don't be a slob. It's fine to sweat profusely, but only if you clean up after yourself and not make others have to share in it.

Use Marijuana to Zone Out

Sometimes using a little ganja is a great way to space out and just go through the motions to get through long routines. It can make the jog while listening to our favorite music seem that much more enjoyable. It can also be the perfect thing to break up that long hike, bike or subway ride.

A little daily exercise as a dose of prevention can go a long way in regards to taking care of your own body. You can never achieve all of that creative potential if you don't give yourself the time to operate. These little changes or routines in your daily life can help keep you in shape whether you're using marijuana or not at the time. While there are many more day-to-day scenarios, the tips found in this chapter should help you to cover other relatable situations that you encounter in your healthy and positive marijuana lifestyle.

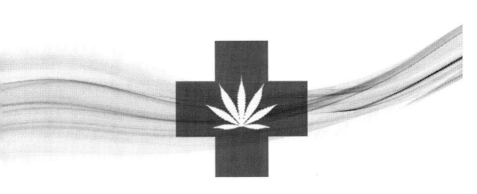

CHAPTER 8

DATING AND MARY JANE

H ere's the ultimate challenge! Balancing romance and Mary Jane. While this topic can surely fill its own book, I'm going to introduce some basic dating concepts that not only have the best odds for success from the beginning when searching for a compatible 420 friendly partner, but also some tips to help avoid letting Mary Jane let your "dream partner" slip through your fingers once you find them.

Make an Informed Choice

If you don't find out some basic things about your potential love interest, you could be setting yourself up for failure right out of the gate. If you know your date even a little bit, you're more likely to build a better foundation for a longer lasting relationship. It's a good decision to find out if the person you are going to consider dating is 420 friendly, or at least how lib-

eral their views are about it. Really pay attention to this: Some
people say anything to get approval during the infatuation
phase of dating, only to try and change the person later, which
inevitably leads to problems. Finding someone you can share
your love of marijuana with is always preferable to someone
who just approves, even if it really doesn't bother him or her
at first. You'd rather be able to smoke with your partner and
enjoy marijuana over the course of a lifetime together.

Once you're on the date, there are some things to keep
in mind so that your love of marijuana doesn't sabotage your
chances with someone special:

- *If you know you can't pull off being high while you're
  on the date, it's probably better not to smoke beforehand.*
  They may be cool that you like marijuana, but
  they probably hope you can stop it for "special"
  occasions, which of course, a first date should be
  to them. Having them wonder how much you *really* smoke is not where you want to be right off
  the bat with your date.
- *Maintain eye contact; don't just rely on body contact.*
  This is just good advice and establishes confidence as well as respect.
- *Cleanliness is next to godliness.* Your date will notice
  everything about your wardrobe and grooming,
  especially those resin stains on your lips, finger-
  nails and jeans. Remember: You *are* being judged
  by your cover.

- *Be prepared to bring your date home.* Do a quick pick up before you leave. Be sure to put away all of your paraphernalia, especially smelly old roaches or gooped up paperclips from cleaning your bowl. Your apartment is where your date is really looking for red flags. They won't be impressed by your collection of 1/8th containers and liquor bottles. Don't get caught off guard and be ready to set the mood, especially if you're planning on blazing together for the first time.

- *Plan fun things to do together that go well with the more cerebral aspects of blazing.* Stimulate your brain while flexing it for your date. Maybe suggest an art gallery or just a nice walk while engaging in a philosophical conversation and perfectly rolled joint. Anyone can get faded and goofy, but here's an opportunity to show how much deeper you are. You're not the "typical" stoner they usually are turned-off to.

- *Be creative and romantic.* Authenticity and honesty can carry you much farther than small talk and a shallow, materialistic conversation. Ultimately this is your time to shine as the modern day sophisticated, intelligent and compassionate marijuana user. If you make sure not to smoke out your potential, your date will be sure to see it too.

Once you've won their heart and most likely had to fib a little
bit about how much you really love marijuana, here are some
ways to possibly smooth the waters and avoid letting marijuana
be the reason that the love of your life slipped through your
fingers.

1. *Try and find someone 420 friendly. This* is the best
   preventative action a Modern Stoner can take. Sharing
   your passion with someone you love is far better than
   having to justify it to them and their circle of friends
   and family on a day-to-day basis.

2. *Always share, but be aware.* Often, it ends up being one
   partner in the relationship who usually supplies the
   green. While this is common, don't be surprised that
   if this is you, you suddenly find the cost of your bud
   has skyrocketed vs. your amount of consumption. This
   is especially true in regards to couples that are heavy
   consumers. Rather than getting furious about your
   partner smoking your entire stash, simply identify your
   combined needs early on, split the costs accordingly
   and divide the bud right when you get it. When you
   toke together, you can both contribute, but if you have
   your own stash, neither one of you has to feel guilty
   or deal with a "Weed Nazi" for a partner. Just having
   this conversation can save a lot of future problems
   between you two. Whenever it applies, it should be
   on the gentleman to at least procure the marijuana
   so that his significant other doesn't need to be in that

position. Depending on where you live, this can be very uncomfortable and the cost can be prohibitive. Rather than get furious about your partner smoking your entire supply, simply split the costs and divide the weed when you get it.

3. *Clean up after yourself.* Do you ever get home after a long day and just want to relax and have your nice little smoke routine? Sometimes, its great to do this with your partner, but usually, we all develop our own little favorite habits during "our time". No one wants to anticipate a nice relaxing night at home and instead, walk into a disaster where your last saved bud has been smoked and your favorite snack eaten. Or maybe you left discarded wrappers everywhere and forgot to record their favorite show? This is *not* a recipe for dating success. To your partner, it just shows that you don't care about their happiness.

4. *Pull your weight with the chores.* Anyone who expects their partner to clean up after them is doomed to be nagged like it's their mother and you end up just wanting to get the hell away from her all over again. Your partner or date isn't there to serve you. You're there to help each other get through life a little easier. Even talking it out makes it easier to maintain a relationship. *Communication is key.*

5. *Vaporize or use edibles if possible.* These methods of using marijuana are not only healthier overall but

lead to increased circulation which translates into better sexual health and a stronger libido. The smell of vaporizing is far cleaner than the burnt smell of a cashed bowl or stale smoke trapped indoors. This can also prevent physical deterioration caused by heavy smoke intake, which keeps people happier with their overall appearance and less likely to have increased insecurity brought on by declined physical health.

6. *Try harder to listen if you are under the influence around your partner.* We all know it's easy to forget stuff when we're smoking herb and while that may get you off the hook every now and then, if you want to be functional day-to-day, you can't always fall back on that excuse. If marijuana inhibits your ability to retain information or focus, then if you want to keep your partner, you have to work harder to listen and remember the information being shared with you. This cannot be stressed enough: *Listening goes a long way.*

7. *Always practice honesty and respect.* Respect your partner's opinions and boundaries on marijuana. Be honest about your use and lifestyle from the beginning of your relationship. If you continue to maintain that honesty, it should help you to find and keep your ideal "threesome". All good relationships are built on a strong foundation and by constant open lines of communication.

8. *Don't internalize your thoughts.* Say them out loud: As much as we all like to think that our partner is psychic, of course, they probably aren't. While your head may be overflowing with genius ideas, if you never verbalize them, you're just stoned, antisocial and kind of boring to be around. Make the conscious effort to vocalize all those crazy thoughts and start up a real conversation together. Isolating yourself when you're high and basically having a conversation in your head to the exclusion of your date—no matter how stimulating it may be to you, is never going to be a success story.

Remember, whether Mary Jane is in the picture or not, dating is just that—dating. The point is to meet partners and try them out for long-term companionship. Simply acquiring years together should not justify reasons to take that next step. Dating is for learning all about your partner and deciding whether or not they are the "compatible crazy" for you, because let's be real, we are all a little crazy in our own way, the trick is finding the person that helps balance us with their craziness day to day. The sooner you identify the right fit for you the better. Typically, the problem lies in people not having the courage or "heart" to make that change right away when their gut tells them for whatever reason this isn't right. If you aren't a good match, sometimes it can drag out forever and waste everyone's time. If marijuana is an important aspect of your life, making sure the person you share it with feels the same way should be important and generally is a better recipe for success.

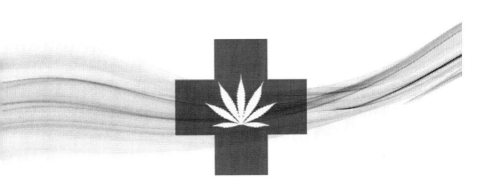

CHAPTER 9

TRAVEL AND R&R

Now that we have balanced marijuana use with our regular day-to-day routines, it's time to take what we've learned and apply it to a vacation or just some well-deserved free time to indulge in some of our favorite sports and activities. In this chapter, I will offer some tips to ensure a great experience when you travel and enjoy your favorite hobbies as a healthy and enlightened marijuana user.

On Your Way...

Whether you travel by trains, planes or automobiles, it's strongly recommended that you know the laws of your destination regarding possession and/or consumption of marijuana. These laws are changing all the time and believe it or not some places still hold some pretty draconian laws, so better to know where they are and if possible avoid them. Until marijuana is reclassified, you are always taking a risk when flying, since it is federal jurisdiction. There have been rumors that TSA has not been enforcing old marijuana laws, but if the wrong TSA agent is in a bad mood on your travel day, it's still within their power to rain hell down on you if they feel like it, regardless of their unofficial new tolerance. Until it's reclassified at a federal level, when push comes to shove, you will always lose. Perhaps it's something to keep in mind next time you're voting. The best idea is to call ahead if you are unsure as some airlines have green-lighted medical marijuana patients ahead of time, providing them with documentation to travel with the herb. Otherwise you will be taking a risk.

Never endanger your fellow travelers by trying to illegally smuggle (or convince your companion) to illegally smuggle marijuana. With marijuana enjoying fairly wide national acceptance, you're likely to find it locally at your destination using only a little ingenuity. You never want to ruin the trip for the group or loved ones because you just "had" to have marijuana. (Edibles may be worth exploring depending on your location in these types of scenarios).

On the Plane...

- **If you're obvious, you should be ready to share.**
  If you're noticeably high (you've become a giddy Chatty Cathy) or brag about it to your seatmate, in certain circumstances you could discreetly offer some of an edible if possible, but be sure to always heed proper warnings before sharing.

However, *it's absolutely unacceptable to incapacitate a fellow traveler.* You have no idea what that person's plans may be on arrival and how you could influence them in a negative way. It would also be a poor introduction to the plant and ruin the edible marijuana experience for them.

- **Be respectful...** not only of physical space, but of other people's audio and olfactory senses. Hmm.... What do we mean? For starters, not everyone wants to be bothered when they are traveling. I'm sure you're super interesting, but everyone has a right to be left alone and not be considered rude for insisting on it.

- **Don't pass gas if you can help it!** Some people believe they can get away with tearing ass because it's hard to peg it to anyone on a packed flight. While this may true, it doesn't make you less of a dirt bag, and while the other passengers may not know the culprit's identity—*you* will.

- **Be mindful of what you bring in regards to your own meal.** Sure you're free to bring whatever food you want. But do you really have to be the person who has the stinky Chinese food that perfectly combines with the crop-dusting mystery funk smell all over the plane to create that special "pre-takeoff aroma" we all associate with air travel?

- **Don't be a slob.** If you're eating and drinking while watching your movie, try your best to get rid of your excess garbage as fast as possible and not spill or leave crumbs on your co passenger. Just talking with your mouth full can be enough to make someone's trip hell.

- **Don't smoke in the bathroom.** Since 9/11, the days when the risk was worth it are long gone. Just wait until you arrive, blaze on the way to the airport or eat an edible beforehand if you can't wait till you get to your destination. You're just asking for major trouble if you light up on board.

In the Car

Although the laws may not be clear, it's in your best interest *not to drive under the influence of marijuana,* regardless of how rational your arguments may seem. Using marijuana in the car is generally a bad habit. So try not to form it. There are some actions to avoid while driving or in other similar situations to avoid letting marijuana become a negative influence in your life. Most of these bad habits can be broken by understanding why they tend to happen and learning how you can avoid them.

Once you've arrived at your destination, whether it was by a long flight or by a short car ride, you want to make sure you aren't left wanting your Mary Jane throughout your travel adventure. Be sure to apply what you've already learned about socializing with friends. There's no "right" or "wrong" way to combine marijuana and your sport; these are simply some guidelines that have helped others along the way. Below, I have listed a few of the most common activities and the ways to make bringing marijuana along a little smoother for you.

Snowboarding/Skiing

To many, snowboarding has become one of the more common sports associated with the younger marijuana culture when it comes to their choice of winter activities. Having the right high while surfing down a mountainside playing the right tunes can be the perfect escape. Given the extreme conditions there a few things you should always be aware of to ensure the smoothest and most enjoyable marijuana experience for yourself and your fellow tokers.

- *It's Best to Toke on the Lift Up.* This must be initiated right after getting on the lift. It's good to pre-roll a blunt for this activity and possibly trim it short by a little less than one quarter, like a ¾ blunt. The reason we want a blunt over a joint is simply because a blunt wrap is more stable in these conditions. It not only prevents canoeing, but it also creates a stronger cherry to survive the cold.

- *It's important to keep the blunt stored in a hard container to protect if from falls* (if you don't get to it on the first run), but not be too large to hurt you if you fall. The container needs to be accessible so you can light it right after you get on the lift and move away from the base.

- *Having a torch lighter filled with butane before you go can save you from frustration.* Your trusty Bic lighter may fail to light due to harsh temperatures, or you could be wasting valuable lift time trying to get the blunt lit in the most likely, windy conditions. The sooner you're lit, the less likely you'll be having to toss any unsmoked herb before you get to the top. Note: *Make sure your gloves are always attached to your wrists before taking them off to handle your blunt and lighter!*

- *Listening to music is amazing while snowboarding or skiing,* but sometimes when you're feeling nice and in the groove, you can't hear the other boarders or skiers shouting their warnings to look out for potential hazards over the loud voices blasting from your ear buds. If you just found some sweet instrumental tunes those warning shouts would pop out a lot more—not to mention it may be a little more soothing. But that's merely my opinion.

Golf

Golf has traditionally been an enjoyable, male-bonding stage for many social or professional events, but women have been increasingly included in the sport and making their presence known. Marijuana has made for a questionable caddy for males and females alike, but ultimately can be a pleasant companion on the course.

- **Does it hurt or help?** This can be up for debate, but the numbers don't lie. Try waiting to toke until you make the turn, and then see if there is a drastic difference between the front or back 9.

- **Splurge on the cart:** A cart gives you the freedom and the privacy to successfully pull off being discreet at the right times and finding the best places for it.

- **Discreet is key:** Golf has always been a little more traditional than other commonly played sports. Generally on the golf course, smoking marijuana—and heavy drinking for that matter, are tolerated, *if you can be civilized about it.*

- **Pre-roll or prepack:** You won't know when your best opportunity to toke will happen, so it's best to be ready when it does.

- **Enjoy the outdoors:** Being able to toke around so much nature is rejuvenating and relaxing.

Team Sports

Choosing the strain is paramount if using marijuana before a game. It's best to choose something more on the Sativa side to keep your energy level up. Because marijuana can affect people in dramatically different ways, it's usually best to save it for the postgame celebration or wound licking. If you find it works well with you personally, find a way to work it into your pregame preparations before you get to the field—unless you can be really stealthy about it. Generally recreational centers frown on marijuana use at the parks. *Never use marijuana around underage children.*

Hiking, Biking & Beach Days

Combining outdoor exercise with Mary Jane is really a staple for the modern day toker. Choosing the right strain is also important for these activities and it's best to lean towards *Sativas* before exercise and *Indicas* to recuperate after. Staying hydrated and packing snacks (always have a backpack) is highly recommended not only to keep your energy levels up but for when the munchies hit as well. The more beautiful the setting, the more amazing the experience! Be prepared for high winds at the beach.

Massage

During a massage, strain selection is also very important. In fact, edibles are possibly the way to experience constant waves of relaxation throughout the massage. Even toking the strongest strain before a 60-minute plus massage is likely to wear off before you get to the end. In this case you may want to lean more towards *Indicas* to help relax the body and ease any discomfort that initially led you to want the massage in the first place.

Water-sports

Protection of the joint is first and foremost if you know you'll be on a boat or around bodies of water. The worst thing you can do is be the one who let the only doob or stash gets washed out and you aren't in the position to just re-up. That can bring on some very disgruntled fellow travelers. Try to add the joint/ stash to your waterproof bag and if possible, put it in its own little doob tube (or small, hard, sealable joint-sized) container.

Group Dinners

If you're arriving with others, a pregame session with some good conversation about food may be a great place to start. Edibles are a fun way to go here. They can be taken prior to the meal and if timed properly, won't kick in until you all arrive at the restaurant. The edible will hit everyone in waves throughout the dinner and you should reap increased effects while enjoying the meal. Knowing what you have already learned about edibles should really help in this scenario. Strain selection may need to be a little more selective. You'll want some of "the munchies" effects, which are usually found in *Indicas*, but without the drag of bringing you and your friends down before the dinner. This is where your own strain research will really pay off so that you can provide the ultimate experience for your guests near every time. *A designated driver is also recommended for these types of outings.*

The social settings that you can bring marijuana into are endless—far too many to cover in this book alone. Warning: It's important to know your boundaries. Never take a chance if you're not sure you can handle the high and the activity at the same time. However, by applying the concepts, tips and information learned throughout this book, you should be well-armed and ready to tackle any social situation with grace and along with an infusion of marijuana you can pull it off with complete success!

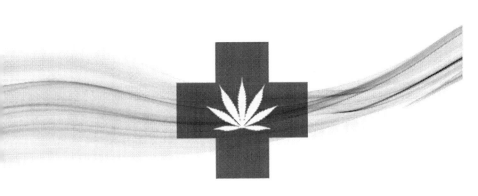

CHAPTER 10

AVOIDING THE DARK SIDE
OF THE SMOKE

While marijuana is arguably the greatest plant to ever be discovered on earth for its medicinal, recreational and industrial applications, it has been shrouded in taboos for decades. While most of these taboos have been fabricated and/or blown out of proportion, sometimes even the most effective lies are woven with a dash of truth. In this chapter, we're going to introduce some concepts to help you and possibly to help others, bypass some of the common problems caused by marijuana abuse.

First, let's talk about one of the most well known "warnings" against marijuana: "*Marijuana is a gateway drug.*" It's an interesting concept: blame a physically non-addictive plant, that's more likely to raise your inhibitions than lower them, for all the other harmful and addictive drugs someone may try. In a way, life itself is a gateway drug and at some time or another *we are all going to be exposed to many things.* You chose marijuana over other drugs because you were making an educated decision to use a safe medicinal *and* recreational plant as an alternative to harmful options such as cigarettes or alcohol, or in place of the addictive pharmaceuticals being dispensed to the nation by our medical professionals.

But now that you've done your research and officially made marijuana your recreational and/or medicinal plant of choice, you have most likely brought it into your daily life. It's important to understand and anticipate that this can lead to changes in attitudes, long-term goals and day-to-day motivations, depending on strain choices and where you are in your life. This can be manifested in dramatically different ways from individual to individual because we're all on our own journey.

In the following pages, I will lay out some concepts to help beginner and seasoned tokers alike avoid falling into some common bad habits or traps that are sometimes all too easy to slip into. Once we come to recognize them, we need to learn what we can do to break them.

Friends and Family

We often end up catching a lot of crap for our newly discovered love of marijuana. Sometimes it's just your drinking buddies missing you or possibly your family not loving all the new things you're into. This can be very annoying and often they don't know what's its like to be you unless they walk a mile in your shoes. But, in the back of your mind, try and let *this* little seed live. Close friends and family may be just the red flag you need to keep an issue from becoming a much bigger problem, and being honest with yourself and with them can help simple concerns from spiraling out of control. Too many times, people can let their defensiveness over smoking herb prevent them from understanding that they probably could be better off making some adjustments, or to become more aware of any changes happening to them as they use marijuana more regularly. Keep in mind that although your family and friends are trying to help, they may well be:

- *Exaggerating:* Sometimes families and friends can blow things way out of proportion. But it's usually based on some truth and they mean well. You can use your extensive knowledge of marijuana to put the minds of your friends and families at ease rather than ignoring and/or isolating yourself. That behavior can only lead to larger problems that from the outside observer's perspective will directly point to your new marijuana use.

- *Don't rely on others or be a burden to others.* You are responsible for yourself and your actions.

- *Know yourself best, and make adjustments.* Your friends and family may come to you with ten things they find they don't like since you started blazing. Maybe nine of them are ridiculous, but that tenth one, you can kind of see. Always be open to the fact that you're getting free feedback about *you*, and if used properly, it can bring on personal improvements. Utilize this but be selective. Above all, be honest. Try not to hate on your loved ones but instead, help them to understand your choice and clear up any misinformation they may have.

Rash Decisions

You may discover a "new" career path is the right thing for you if you now find yourself unhappy in your current job or school. Seeking out something more in line with the "new" you, although it may be entirely different, may be the better direction. But keep in mind, it can be daunting and it's generally better to line up a new job or school *first* before making a drastic decision—no matter how right it *seems*. There's a real risk of being cut short financially, leaving you with ample time to be lured into bad habits with marijuana, and ultimately less spending money for it too.

Trading Places

Avoid trading favorite hobbies for couch time with your new friend Mary Jane. Don't lose the other things you love in your life because you'd rather smoke marijuana. Instead, find ways to incorporate them *both*. The best way is to find strains that compliment the activity you're doing as we spoke about in great depth in earlier chapters (e.g. *Know Your Meds*). It's not a bad thing if you find some of your interests changing as you begin to use marijuana, but make sure that if you're going to trade in one of your old hobbies, *first* you find something new to replace it so you don't end up having lots of downtime and getting in the comfortable routine of chilling on the couch all day. It's like staying home from work or school too long; eventually you never want to go back and it becomes that much harder. Try and do at least one physical activity a week at the minimum. And stay active!

Commitment to Hygiene

Avoid letting up on regular grooming. You already know how to incorporate the messy/beach look and make it look sharp if that's what you're going for. But just doing it once doesn't cut it. Sometimes time seems to fly a little faster when you start with regular marijuana use and those haircut and nail appointments may become further and further apart. Stay on top of it! It keeps you feeling fresh and keeps people from assuming the worst, which we already know they do.

Mary Jane vs. Martha Stewart

Avoid redecorating your home with Mary Jane paraphernalia. There are many ways to express your enjoyment without having to set yourself back with parents or potential partners. There are much better ways to show you appreciate the herb than to beat people over the head with memorabilia. It also looks completely juvenile. I'm not saying you shouldn't represent, but do it with class and choose items that have special meaning to you.

Marijuana should *lead* to creative forms of expression, not *be* your creative form of expression.

Time after Time

Avoid becoming a flaky stoner slacker. Your friends and family will pick up on this first and then target your sweet smelling girl Mary Jane second. Flaking on people is the fast track to taking heat for smoking herb. Keeping your word and appointments is a quality valued by many people and for better or for worse; it follows you around throughout your life. You never know when your word will be all you have. If you're having trouble getting out the door or remembering appointments or plans, try setting reminders on your phone or just alarms in general. Sometimes you have to go a little out of your way to prevent messing up, but in the end, isn't setting an alarm worth preventing fallouts from annoyed friends and family? More than likely, they'll end up blaming your new "buds" for your flaky behavior. Marking down birthdays and anniversaries on a wall or desk calendar can really help too. Just sit down one day with your favorite strain and knock it out. Splurge the few bucks on a calendar and take a blazed afternoon and you can avoid being the stoner who always forgets birthdays. With social media these days, who really has an excuse?

"High" Me vs. "Sober" Me

Find a balance sooner than later. When you first start to smoke, it's normal to start to challenge some of your previously held ideas. Before you make any drastic decisions, it's always best to think things out. As you get more comfortable with using marijuana, your two sides *should* eventually merge, usually through compromise. If you have trouble with your "high self" messing up things for your "sober self", it's best to use marijuana as a relaxation tool and not a tool for making life decisions. If you're not sure what you want to do with your life yet, marijuana can be a blessing or a curse. Sometimes the longer you take to figure it out, you might feel guilty for your marijuana use. It's common for people to temporarily escape their reality using heavier marijuana strains to avoid making those types of life decisions. While it's still the safest choice for doing so, it is not recommended. Time waits for no one—whether you smoke marijuana or not. *Marijuana shouldn't hold you back, but be a helpful companion on your journey.*

Express Yourself

Avoid shutting down. Sometimes writing or saying your conflicting thoughts out loud can help clarify things for you. If you begin feeling lost, you would be surprised what just a 2 day break can do for you, not only for clarity of mind, but for easing any possible brewing thoughts that you *need* marijuana. Daily use may not be the best thing for you if you are finding it difficult to balance a positive healthy lifestyle. It's quite possible that after you find your stride in life, marijuana may be better suited for you to help safely alleviate daily stresses or for medicinal benefits.

A Righteous Bore

Avoid being the guy who "just found religion" and needs to beat everyone over the head with it. *"Marijuana is awesome!! How have you never known this before?"* Keep in mind that millions if not billions *have* in some way, shape or form before you, discovered marijuana and they might just know something you don't, so be respectful of others as well as those who have not "seen the light" yet. Always be willing to share knowledge in a non-combative and easygoing way. Be willing to back off if someone seems uninterested or has opposing feelings on the subject. Always be willing to listen and then intelligently debate the subject but never be condescending or talk down to someone who has less knowledge.

Stay Healthy and Fit

Avoid feelings of depression from seeing and feeling the physical effects of smoking. Aging is already difficult enough. While marijuana smoke is not as harmful as cigarette smoke in any fashion, and as a former heavy cigarette smoker for over ten years and an even heavier marijuana smoker for the next 10 years after that, I can tell you that there are some slight similarities. What can you do? First, I would recommend converting to vaporizing ASAP. If getting more potency isn't enough for you, it may help to lift that unhealthy glow about you in the mirror. Why? Well for one, the smoke isn't really good for your skin—*or* your hair for that matter. It can lead to premature thinning and balding and/or dry skin. Poor circulation also leads to dampening your appearance and likely lowered libido. Edibles are the other way to go here to take the occasional break from the smoke and still be left satisfied. Utilize what you've learned about edibles to make sure you're not left wanting more *or* wanting to get it out of you ASAP.

Remember to Brush

Avoid unnecessary dental problems. Dentists are extremely expensive and a session with one can be very, very painful. Enter the late night junk food binges, waking up in the middle of the night on the couch, credits rolling with all the lights on…not knowing how it happened. Most likely brushing won't be your first stop on your way to bed. Be sure to get or stay in the habit of brushing and flossing your teeth before you go to sleep. Stoners end up suffering from a lot of dental issues and it's no coincidence that dentists pop up at the cannabis cups and hemp conventions.

You Have A Friend

Getting random marijuana strains without knowing the genetics and effects or without access to the information to help sort it out for yourself can make the "marijuana name game" a major problem for many people. If you live in areas where legal forms of marijuana are available to you, make sure you feel good about from whom and where you are getting your strains and edibles. If you don't have many options, try and shop around and when you find something you like, buy it in bulk. But be sure to know your local laws and take proper precautions.

Only the Best!

Avoid choosing only the heaviest strains to a fault. Don't burn yourself out! Changes in energy levels, appetite, weight and attitude can be linked to changing strains and if you are aware of your general behavior even week to week, you can avoid any negative irregularities from becoming habit forming. Remember, it's not a competition of who can smoke the *strongest* strains. The challenge is finding the strains that are the *perfect balance for you* throughout your day.

Avoid Boasting

One, no one wants to feel inferior or pressured in social situations, and two, most likely you are just creating a brand (the *"Cheech"* or *"Chong"* of your group) for yourself amongst your friends by bragging about how much *more* than everyone else you toke. They'll remember all too well, don't worry.

Avoid Smoking in Public Areas (But if you can't—be discreet!)

Generally being discreet is always the desirable tactic here. But keep in mind sometimes just out of sight isn't out of mind. Using edibles can simply avoid problems altogether, but in certain areas, safe consistent edibles can still be hard to find, or not exist at all yet, even in our most popular urban environments. In these cases we are generally left to smoking it somehow. While we already discussed the pros and cons of various methods, you still need to keep in mind that the smell is what you need to mask the most and is most likely to give you away.

Some other things to keep in mind:

- If you smoke around parents with children, mothers with baby, school zones and other clearly marked drug free zones... you are asking for it! Most police today are less prone to strict enforcement of marijuana laws due to its decriminalization in many states. This doesn't mean they *can't* or *won't* enforce it if necessary; but typically, most cops don't want to hassle with the paperwork preferring to focus on bigger issues. However, if Joe Citizen goes to the police and reports that you are openly smoking pot in the neighborhood, be prepared to be busted! That's on you for not knowing better.
- Avoid the coughing fits. Bring water; just the slightest coating on the throat can help.
- Have everything ready to go so you aren't visibly rolling or packing.

If Possible, Avoid Buying Illegally

Unfortunately we live in a world where marijuana is still criminalized in most places. Therefore it can be difficult to obtain. If you have no choice and are not willing to move to a more 420 friendly state, than here are some things you should keep in mind:

- You never know what an illegal street dealer is involved in. Every time you're interacting with them, you are putting yourself into their world and exposing yourself to some of their risks.

- There's much more diversity in choice and higher quality grade marijuana available in legal or medicinal markets.

- Don't get ripped off, even if your options are limited. Thanks to pioneers in the industry putting good information out there, you can still be a fairly educated consumer when navigating the darker, more illegal marijuana markets. Unfortunately, sometimes we have no choice but to pay extra for the unavailability, and the reality of "It's better than nothing at all" must be seriously entertained *before* you get too picky.

The Company We Keep

Identify "Moochers." You should always understand that misery loves company and generally won't push you out. Knowing who your real friends are can really help you avoid surrounding yourself with negative enablers. Often, they're the true "gateway drug." Know what you want and surround yourself with like-minded people. If you let yourself drift, there's no telling what types of people you may let into your life who could have hazardous effects on many aspects of it. If they always "just wanna chill" and never really do or build towards anything, then they're not the type of creative "tokers" you want to be around. These people exist in all walks of life and a certain percentage of people will abuse anyone and anything they can. Don't let that be an excuse or let that be the reason you fall into an unmotivated slacker state. Know who you are and what you want. Don't compromise your values or lifestyle choice in exchange for mooching company. If you don't know what you want, there'll always be someone who will try and decide for you. On the flip side, there are others like *you*, who can be motivated, ambitious and creative while blazing at the same time. You just need to find them, but they are out there—in numbers!

Don't be a "Mooch" Yourself!

Sure it's hard to pass up a hit of Mary Jane on any occasion, especially if you find yourself amongst a cool group of communal tokers. It's important to give back to this seemingly selfless supply of marijuana that's flowing in your direction. It all works sort of like Karma, and people will notice if the smoke always seems to flow in one direction. You never want to be "The Mooch." By the time you have to be called out for it, it's too late and now you'll be obliged to go out of your way to prove you're not a moocher. Being stingy in the short-term will probably cost you *more* in the long run.

Don't Tell People Where You Grow or Stash Your Grass!

I know it can be very tempting to show off your green thumb or all the varieties of buds you have, but keep in mind, if you don't *really* know the people you're with, they may very likely be thinking about how they can make *your* stuff *their* stuff. It's sad but true. Even if you do trust all your friends or family members, they may be so impressed or blown away with your setup or stash they can't help but gossip to all *their* friends about it. *Their* friends may not have the same discretion about your stuff as they do and that information can later become, "Hey I heard about this place nearby that has a lot of plants and no security!" Take pictures and never disclose locations!

Generally Avoid Blazing at School or Work

Unfortunately, our society has not evolved to the point to understand that a bunch of students sitting in a field sharing a joint discussing politics or philosophy is not more dangerous to the learning environment than keg stands, Adderall cramming and chain-smoking to deal with stresses. Until common sense is employed on a massive scale, be sure not to burn past, present or future bridges in regards to work or school by burning marijuana against the rules.

Avoid Toking before or While Studying or before / during / in between Classes

It's important to understand that there are components of marijuana designed to help us forget more irrelevant information in our daily lives; this is so our brain doesn't overload on information. In certain settings this can be frustrating, or worse, it can lead to having problems performing in our day-to-day tasks. If you're a student of any kind, it's important to pay attention and monitor your grades and performance as you begin to introduce marijuana more thoroughly throughout your daily activities. On the contrary, it's possible you find marijuana and studying merge well with you. That's fine too. The key is monitoring and being honest while making changes when necessary. You must be honest with yourself and take note when negative trends begin to form, such as slipping grades, angry friends and family etc. If you find you're having trouble focusing, or you feel like you're slipping or stuck in a rut, here are few ideas to try and bring you back:

- *Let up on the usage or even take a break* to clear up and establish your goal and what you need to change.

- *Set your goals, and then set up shop.* Soberly set the precedence for the habits you want to have when you study and then slowly introduce marijuana after a few successful trial runs.

- *Use a reward system.* You may find that toking *while* you do most of your daily activities or going to the gym really helps get through it; most people find that when studying information, especially when it is not information the person is passionate about, is very difficult to retain. In this case, it's better to use marijuana as a reward system. Study and get through your work. Once you're satisfied with the completed project or at least the checkpoint you set for yourself, reward yourself with a nice toke break. Only *you* know what is best for *you,* and only you will suffer from not being honest with yourself. Sometimes studying for concepts rather than just rote-memorizing information can be helpful also.

Proofread, Proofread, and Proofread!

Today, we're able to hide behind many types of communication to cater to a few of the anti-social effects that *daily* marijuana use can sometimes lead to. We really have no excuse for presenting ourselves online in a sloppy manner. Using automated tools such as "spellcheck" to proofread emails and texts can go a long way in how people perceive your digital image. The question for the recipient becomes: if you write like you're illiterate, will you talk and act like that too?

Don't Toke, Drink and Drive

Try to avoid driving while just starting to smoke herb, and generally thereafter. Most of the terrible statistics released about smoking marijuana and driving are *drastically reduced* when you *remove the alcohol* use from them. In most cases, many of those marijuana related accident cases were actually people who were under the influence of alcohol, but also tested positive for marijuana use in their blood, which still doesn't guarantee that it was used at the time of the incident.

Avoid Smoking and Driving Simultaneously

It's hard to tell how you will adjust to the marijuana high *as* you are smoking. Sometimes this makes it much more difficult to drive. It only takes one mistake and one bad adjustment for something lifelong or worse, life-ending, to happen in an instant.

Avoid Selling Marijuana Illegally

Many people fall in to the trap of selling marijuana on the

black market for a variety of reasons. It can give them free head smoke or dramatically bring their cost of bud down. It provides a seemingly easy job with the illusion of big money simply because it deals in cash. But always keep in mind:

- It creates short-term money but long term problems.

- It's a tempting gig for couch potato. What's easier than sitting on your butt all day selling someone else's bud for a nominal kickback on the black market? Probably sitting on your butt in a prison cell, so at least you'll be well trained.

- It's easy for a friend's acquaintance/dealer to rat you out. You may be smooth, but do you trust every single person you're selling to not sell you down the river at the first sign of their freedom being taken away? If your answer is yes, you'll learn the error of your ways *while you're serving their time.* Never forget that you're the "get out of jail free card" for everyone you sell to.

Realistically, in today's world if you just *have* to work in marijuana there are over 21 states you can do so legally. People have moved from all over the country and the world to get in on the beginning of the booming legal marijuana market. Often they have had their battles. Selling marijuana in an illegal state on principle, or just thinking you're too smart to get caught, is a one-way ticket to disaster. Luckily, there are many legal ways to thrive within the marijuana culture and we truly stand at the precipice of an enormous developing industry.

Avoid Carrying Large Amounts of MJ on Your Person

There are limited situations when this could be necessary. Generally, you shouldn't need more than 1/8th on your person at any given time. The more you carry, the more you raise the suspicion of being an illegal dealer. This can draw a whole different level of attention from the police as opposed to just the average user with possession. *Selling marijuana illegally has not been decriminalized in most places and you should avoid suspicion at all costs.*

Think about the risks you take if you become involved in any of the actions I have listed in this chapter. Are they really worth it? Remember, in the world of marijuana, you may often be right and rational but that doesn't always matter to the outside world. Now that you understand the game and how to play it, you have greatly increased your chances to survive and prosper in this overly judgmental society. *Always* consider the risk vs. the rewards. Remember, there are ways to incorporate marijuana discreetly into anything you do. The key is to find the right balance for you!

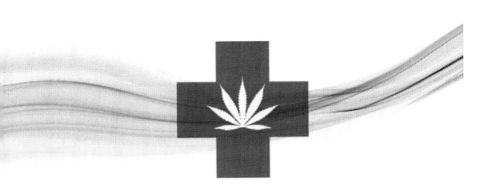

CONCLUSION

BALANCING THE MARY JANE LIFE

Balancing a healthy, modern marijuana lifestyle will always be a work in progress and may prove to be challenging for you at first, but one of the best aspects of toking marijuana with others is the tolerant vibe and many rewards that come with it. Throughout my book, I have outlined a few good concepts to inhale that will ensure that you'll be able to maintain that positive vibe with others and make your place in the world a positive one.

Sharing is truly caring, and in the end, we all live on this planet just trying to make a happy life for ourselves and to make sense of our complex existence. At our core, that's who we are. The less we try and fool ourselves and other people that we've got it all figured out, the more easily we can see how similar we all are and learn from each other. Your honesty can bring tolerance and compromise.

While the marijuana culture is one that should be cherished and when possible, shared with others, many people believe in or place value on different types of things. Just as they have no right to mock you, your beliefs or behavior, in return, you shouldn't mock others for being different or just because they fail to see your point of view—regardless of how "ridiculous" they may seem to you. By opening an intelligent debate, if nothing else, both sides may actually *learn something*! Actually, the best way to argue your point is to *not argue at all*, but rather *explain* your idea kindly, clearly and confidently. If you can get someone to understand *why* you say something, you have a much better chance of getting them to *see it* from your point of view more clearly. If you expect someone to take your point seriously you should be prepared to be able to fully explain your logic. Articulate clearly and kindly, and be sure not to be judgmental or condescending. Making your point like an a-hole and making someone feel stupid is not in the spirit of sharing the marijuana lifestyle.

Live and Let Live

Simply put, what a person wants from life varies between every individual on the planet. Our understanding of the world and feeling of our place and purpose can vary dramatically and come in all shapes and sizes. The world is full of endless combinations of ways to spend your life depending on what your soul is craving. Based on *your* personal journey to this point, what *your* soul craves will inevitably be different from the other souls sharing the planet. The modern, enlightened marijuana user will always be respectful of that.

If you find enjoyment in some of life's little treasures, leave it there for someone else to enjoy as well. If you find a problem, be the solution rather than just complain about it. At the minimum, clean up after yourself and be mindful of your carbon footprint.

Defending yourself and your marijuana lifestyle to a fault can be very harmful to both your personal and work relationships. After all, who are you really helping? When you have to, by all means stand your ground, but if you're just good at debate and winning arguments (which doesn't mean you're always right by the way) beware: You may win the argument, but you still lose every day that you maintain your bad habit. Take criticism constructively and know the difference between "haters" and "helpers" in your life.

What Goes Around Comes Around

Although it's arguably one of the truest concepts floating through our existence, that simple statement is misleading as to its potentially immeasurable, cosmic implications. People often say, "Karma's a bitch", but that's always in reference to people doing negative, harmful acts to others and having it come back to kick them in the ass. In theory, it does work both ways: by exercising kindness and good Karma, you'll receive good Karma back. How immediate it may be has a lot to do with how backed-up your Karmatic slate may be.

Scrubbing the slate clean by coming clean about old lies

and removing negative inputs/outputs from your life can be instrumental in speeding up your good Karma. On the flip side, if you just keep getting hit with wave after wave of bad luck, you might be atoning for multiple years' worth of high school or college bad behavior, cheating on partners or screwing people over (only you know the truth). The sooner you stop that bleeding, the sooner you should see positive change coming back into your life. Be proactive! Seek out people you've wronged and make it right. You could be blown away at how your life can change.

As you move forward on the path to building a healthy marijuana lifestyle as I have described in the preceding chapters, remember—*there's no money in curing a disease, but there is billions in treating one.* This is scary, but a commonly accepted reality in medicine nowadays. First, people are generally prescribed medicine to treat an illness. Then *sometimes* the illness is successfully suppressed, yet can cause multiple other "side effects" that now need to be treated—so you're prescribed more meds to treat the "side effects" from the meds you got to treat the initial illness. In many cases, the combinations of these meds, while also costly (or profitable, depending on which side of it you're on) end up causing more problems and/or not achieving its intended therapeutic effect. They can burn out major organs, lead to fatalities due to overdose, medication error, or long-term wear and tear from abuse. As you begin to look into how these meds make it to the market, the lack of health regulation on them, the blatant "marketing" money being spent on promoting them and compliant doctors to prescribe them, you may get a better perspective on how your health is being monetized. Always do your research when it comes to your health and health of your loved ones; in this economy is it really unimaginable to think doctors could be corrupted by bribes or perks fuelled by a billion-dollar pharmaceutical industry?

Now that you're well on your way to becoming an enlightened member of the marijuana world, you're responsible to be aware of your limits—*then* push yourself slightly past them little by little. How well you handle yourself in light of knowing your boundaries can help you prevent many undesirable situations. Becoming all the things you want rarely happens overnight and it can all seem like a long and daunting path ahead. Think big and execute small. Start with one little thing outside of your comfort zone and let it lead you gently into your unknown. Be confident. You'll get to where you need to be. The first step is starting to move.

Remember that using only one type of strain is like reading one page from the greatest book ever written. Hold on to what you love, but be open to trying new things, not only in marijuana, but life in general. The sooner you find out what you want from life, the sooner you can take action and make progress towards achieving it. Until then, there will *always* be someone who knows what you should do. It's best to keep in mind that these people are often more interested in *how you can best help them to achieve what they want* rather than a genuine interest or concern for you. Armed with the information, tips and concepts I have provided, always be prepared to take accountability for your actions and go into the world open-minded. We'll all be faced with a variety of opportunities and choices throughout our lifetime. Just be mindful that these choices, for better or worse, can have short or long-term effects far greater than we initially anticipate—not only for ourselves, but also for the lives of others around us. Marijuana should *lead to* creative forms of expression and not *be* your creative form of expression.

As much as I hope you have enjoyed this book and can take away lots of useful information, there is no absolute, "money-back-guarantee" guidebook for life. No one knows *all* the answers and no one knows the truth about the existence or non-existence of God, not even His Holiness, the Pope, himself.

The only consistent thing in life is change.

At some point in human history, every man-made thing you see around you and nearly every job you can think of probably didn't exist. So it begs the question, "What is life really about on this planet?" Of course, no one can answer that for you, but for me, one thing is for sure: I'd rather have Mary Jane with me for the ride while I try and figure it out.

It's my sincere hope that I've helped you to discover the modern, healthy, and positive ways to *safely* and *enjoyably* keep marijuana in your life while maximizing your potential and finding your special place in the world!

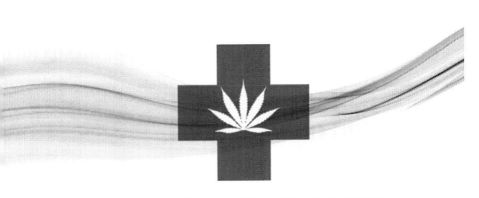

ACKNOWLEDGMENTS

A special thank you to—

- My parents, Karen & Bob and Charles & Grace: for always keeping an open mind and trusting in my choices.

- Caterina, my true soul mate: Thank you for all your love and support, and for always challenging my ideas and perspective. You make me believe that anything is possible!

- Danny Reed: Thank you for believing in my vision from day 1 to bring truth to patients, and for your unwavering dedication to expose the injustices of the marijuana industry. Your research and insight has been invaluable over the years.

- My team at the Root Cellar, Los Angeles: You guys bring these words to life and share them every day—Donald Harwell, Heather Fix, Nick Nehring, Eve Modens, Russell Knight and Lauren Hanley.

- Brian (with an "i") Albert: Your experience and good-natured kindness throughout the marijuana community has brought marijuana into many lives in a positive, non-judgmental way.

- Tommy, my positive enabler! Thank you for believing.

- Dr. Jeffrey C. Raber, Phd, University Southern California (The Werc Shop Independent Laboratory): Thank you for offering truth in testing and providing a bright light in the otherwise dark age of modern marijuana research (http://thewercshop.com). Your selflessness in sharing knowledge for the greater good of medicinal and recreational marijuana consumers has been both an inspiration and a catalyst to change.

- Lynne D. Scott, my kick-ass editor: There are no words....

- David Dunham, Joel Dunham and The Dunham Group: Thank you for getting it and seeing my vision. Your guidance and contributions in helping me to achieve my dream are deeply appreciated.

- And finally... to the great patients at the Root Cellar and everyone I've shared a toke with over the years: The many experiences I've had with all of you has led me to write this book to share my ideas for a positive and enlightened marijuana lifestyle. I wish only the happiest and healthiest relationship for you and marijuana throughout your life.

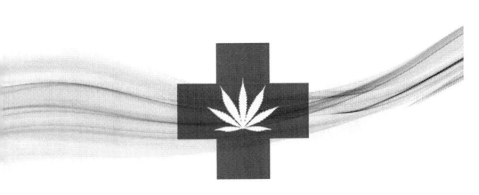

ABOUT THE AUTHOR

Michael Green often identifies himself as "a serial entrepreneur." He began studying at John Jay College of Criminal Justice for a career in federal law enforcement, changed course to travel and to teach English in Prague, Barcelona and Budapest, before establishing a number of successful start-ups in both the marijuana and non-marijuana fields. Michael is currently the owner and operator of a successful medical marijuana dispensary in Los Angeles along with multiple news, media and information web properties. He is dedicated to bringing consumer awareness and promoting responsible marijuana etiquette to the community. Effectively balancing his many ventures while maintaining a more than average daily marijuana use, Michael Green is a real-life example of *Modern Marijuana Living*.

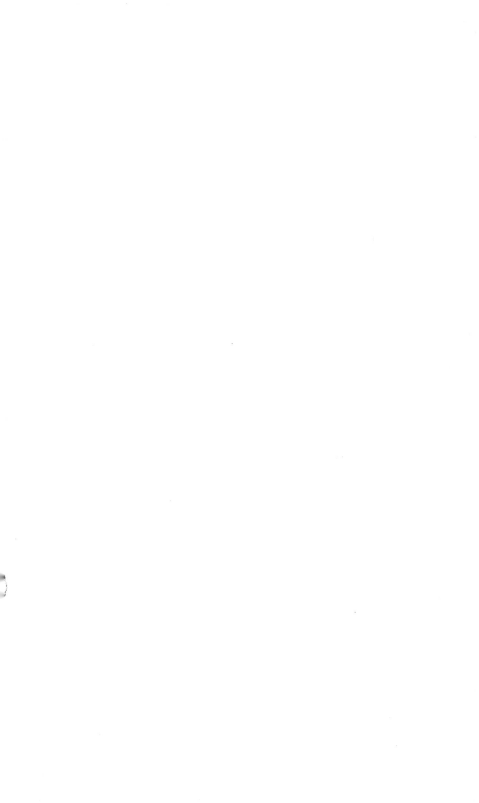